Global Health Leadership

Mellissa Withers • Judith McCool
Editors

Global Health Leadership

Case Studies from the Asia-Pacific

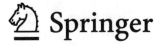 Springer

Editors
Mellissa Withers
Keck School of Medicine
USC Institute for Global Health
Los Angeles, CA, USA

Judith McCool
School of Population Health
University of Auckland
Auckland, New Zealand

ISBN 978-3-319-95632-9   ISBN 978-3-319-95633-6   (eBook)
https://doi.org/10.1007/978-3-319-95633-6

Library of Congress Control Number: 2018955903

This Springer imprint is published by the registered company Springer Nature Switzerland AG
The registered company address is: Gewerbestrasse 11, 6330 Cham, Switzerland

Foreword

The societies bordering the Pacific Ocean make up over one-third of the world's population and around 60% of global GDP and 47% of global trade. They are highly diverse in terms of culture, language, health and education infrastructure, economic well-being, physical environment, and political participation—and thus in their ability to manage human health challenges from natural disasters to disease.

Situated around the world's largest ocean covering more than one-third of the world's surface, Pacific Rim societies on the "Ring of Fire" dominate geophysical events statistics both in terms of exposed population and of infrastructure. The Asia-Pacific region also accounts for 40% of the world's natural disaster events, nearly 60% of global disaster deaths and 80% of storm mortality worldwide.[1] Seventy percent of air pollution deaths occur in the Asia-Pacific region. Chemical production in the region is projected to increase by 46% between 2012 and 2020, and the region is estimated to produce 1 million tons of hazardous waste daily.

The region is also home to wide disparities in life expectancy and in the capacity to meet the challenges of climate change, disasters, and disease burdens. These are a few of the most obvious indicators of the connectivity between the health of the planet and human health around the Pacific Rim. Hence, the need exists for the comprehensive understanding of health, which drives APRU's Global Health Program.

This book is unique not only for the diversity of the societies it covers but also for the range of disciplines of the international specialists who authored the case studies and bring their vision, leadership, cultural competency, and analytical abilities to global health challenges. The topics of the case studies range from tobacco control and noncommunicable diseases to maternal health services and disaster preparedness. Each case draws from academics, researchers, and global health leaders at the forefront of interdisciplinary research in the Asia-Pacific region. The examination of cases from different countries and sectors includes input from private corporations, governments, communities, NGOs, and multilateral

---

[1] APRU Impact Report 2016.

organizations. As this book is intended as a learning resource, each chapter includes discussion questions and recommended readings.

APRU is uniquely positioned to promote global health. Its 50 members are leading research universities representing a significant proportion of the research and education capabilities of the APEC economies, linking the research and professional communities of the Americas, Asia, and Australasia. As the voice of knowledge and innovation for the region, we bring together thought leaders, researchers, and policy-makers to exchange ideas and collaborate on effective solutions to twenty-first-century challenges. The APRU Global Health Program and this book are perfect illustrations of this.

We recognize the need for a new level of connectivity and cooperation to address the disparity between societies which have high capacity in global health and those where the burden of disaster and disease is greatest. The Global Health Program, now in its 11th year, has shown results in more efficient use of resources, greater consistency in standards and methods, improved outcomes and impact, while helping to ease the burden of interventions for regulatory authorities. For our member universities, the chance to work with external partners has given them access to new pools of knowledge and helped save on research and development costs.

Universities have a unique and crucial role to play in terms of the promotion of health and well-being of populations now and in the future. Not only do they generate ideas and provide evidence-based solutions and academic leadership, they also prepare tomorrow's global health professionals for challenges yet unknown. This role is now more important than ever, as rapid changes in demographics and the environment are accelerating the propagation of global health challenges. Fast-footed, effective networks of collaboration and professional trust will be more important than ever.

This book is intended as a resource in the broader endeavor to exchange professional experience, encourage cooperation across borders of all kinds, and to inform public policy at all levels.

Association of Pacific Rim Universities   Christopher Tremewan
Clear Water Bay, Hong Kong

Preface

Our global interdependence and collective exposure to transnational threats to population health and well-being are becoming increasingly apparent. As the world and its economies become globalized, in part due to extensive international mobility and commerce, the need to address health in a global context has become essential. Many of the pressing global health concerns are shared problems requiring collaborative solutions. Global phenomena such as aging, urbanization, migration, environmental degradation, natural disasters, and rising rates of noncommunicable diseases transcend geographical boundaries and cultures.

This book introduces students to the various models and practice of leadership in the field of global health from the Pacific Rim region through problem-based learning. We bring together an interdisciplinary group of academics, researchers, and leaders from around the world who are conducting innovative programs and high-quality research in the field of global health. This timely book provides an overview of the challenges in global health leadership from multiple perspectives, illustrating theoretical and conceptual ideas of leadership through case studies of successful global health interventions.

The field of global health is defined as "... an area for study, research, and practice that places a priority on improving health and achieving health equity for all people worldwide" (Koplan et al., 2009[1]). Solutions to current and future global health challenges will require collaboration from a specialized workforce from many disciplines and sectors. International agencies such as the World Health Organization, local and national governments, nongovernmental organizations, community leaders, and the private sectors all have key leadership roles to play in developing, implementing, and evaluating programs that promote health and well-being. With disparities in health outcomes, both within and between countries, now greater than at any time in recent history, leaders skilled to respond to these global health challenges are indispensable. This book highlights important elements

---

[1] Koplan, J. P., Bond, T. C., Merson, M. H., et al. (2009). For the Consortium of Universities for Global Health Executive Board. Towards a common definition of global health. Lancet, 373, 1993–1995.

in global health leadership, including cooperation, problem solving, vision, social justice, and cultural competency.

More than 40 economies belong to the diverse Pacific Rim region, representing Asia, Australia and Oceania, and the Americas. This book includes case studies from Australia, Indonesia, Japan, Malaysia, the Pacific Islands, New Zealand, the Philippines, South Korea, the United States, and Vietnam. Despite obvious political, economic, social, and cultural diversity among countries in the region, disease risk and mitigation factors are shared and typically involve collective action at all levels of governance. Examples of action from grassroots advocacy to whole-of-government leadership are examined in this book.

Learning Objectives

This book will help students to:

1. Identify key trends and issues working in global health contexts
2. Analyze the ways public health, health, systems and other organizations can work together to impact health outcomes
3. Discuss the ways that diverse perspectives may influence policies, programs, services, and the health of a community
4. Explain the need for partnerships in developing, implementing, and evaluating policies, programs, and services that affect the health of a community
5. Identify key characteristics of effective global health leaders
6. Articulate ways to identify and measure success in leadership
7. Describe the challenges faced in health programming and how they were overcome

The tremendous gains in life expectancy witnessed during the twentieth century largely resulted from improvements in living conditions and reductions in infectious disease mortality, leading to increased child survival. While there is still work to be done in terms of child mortality and infectious disease prevention globally, the most serious threats to health and well-being over the next century will undoubtedly come from environmental degradation and rising noncommunicable diseases, including mental health issues. In 2016, the United Nations introduced the Sustainable Development Goals (SDGs), a set of 17 goals and 169 targets designed to help countries mobilize efforts to end poverty, protect the planet, and ensure prosperity. The SDGs encourage the use of these goals to address inequalities and help ensure sustainable social and economic development through collective action. The targets provide specific, measurable objectives on a range of issues, including poverty, infectious diseases, Non-Communicable Diseases (NCDs), gender inequality, education, and climate change. Indeed, Goal #17 relates specifically to partnership and calls for a revitalized and enhanced global partnership that brings together leaders from multiple stakeholders. A stronger commitment to partnership, cooperation, and developing effective leaders that represent diverse communities is required to achieve the ambitious goals set forth in the SDGs.

Leadership has become a key component in graduate-level education and training in global health. Effective leaders do not inherently possess the required characteristics and skills but benefit from leadership training and skill building, reflective practice, and exposure to the complexity of global health issues, which helps to prepare them to respond with compassion, intelligence, and purpose. Given that global health practice is typically conducted in team settings with members from various countries, backgrounds, and cultural contexts, this book also provides students with an opportunity to examine multiple examples of leadership in different contexts. With globalization, most global health organizations are now operating in multicultural environments.

Case studies are increasingly being used to examine the practical application of the theories and skills discussed in leadership courses. They are useful in assisting students in developing problem solving and analytical skills. They help to illustrate complex situations in which the solution is not always straightforward. This book helps students examine global health challenges from multiple perspectives and to analyze decision-making processes and different cultural interpretations of solutions. The operationalization of leadership may differ widely from culture to culture. Case studies have a role in building an appreciation for what constitutes effective leadership within global health and how this may differ by culture or perspective. For example, authority and autocratic leadership is preferred in some cultures while egalitarianism, teamwork, and collaborative decision-making valued in others. We hope that this book promotes discussions around which traits are most important in successful leaders. Innovation, vision, and having the ability to inspire others are almost universally recognized as key leadership characteristics. But do effective leaders also have to be diplomatic, adaptable, friendly, risk-takers, or team players? Variability in leadership styles and preferences for leadership approaches in different cultural contexts are illustrated in this book.

The case studies represented in this book highlight successful examples of leadership from communities, nongovernmental organization, private industries, and local and national governments. Students will learn how leaders have overcome challenges faced in the operationalization of complex health interventions, foreign policy, and working with key stakeholders and organizations in this context. Each chapter includes questions designed to spark conversation, debate, and thought, as well as some additional recommended readings. We encourage examination of the applicability of solutions from one case to other settings and problems.

We also wish to acknowledge that a range of important challenges are not included in this book but are worth mentioning because of their special relevance in the Pacific Rim region. These include natural and man-made disasters, environmental degradation, emerging and reemerging infectious diseases, and reproductive health. While they were beyond the scope of this book, we do not want to diminish their importance in shaping the health of populations around the region and the world.

Despite differences in terms of government structure, health systems, cultural contexts, and available resources, the economies in the Pacific Rim share a similar vision of improved health and well-being among populations in the region, as well as globally. The cases present an opportunity to examine how major health challenges have been addressed based on direct experiences of those at the forefront of global health leadership.

Los Angeles, CA, USA   Mellissa Withers

Acknowledgments

First, we wish to acknowledge the leadership of the four university presidents who founded the Association of Pacific Rim Universities (APRU), whose extraordinary vision and spirit of collaboration brought together thought leaders, researchers, and policy-makers to exchange ideas and collaborate on effective solutions to the challenges of the twenty-first century. They are Thomas Everhart of California Institute of Technology; Chang-Lin Tien of the University of California, Berkeley; Charles Young of the University of California, Los Angeles; and Steven B. Sample of the University of Southern California.

We would also like to thank the leadership of current APRU International Secretariat for their inspiration and dedication to cultivating effective leaders, including Christopher Tremewan (Secretary General) and Christina Schönleber (Director, Policy and Programs). The University of Southern California hosts the APRU Global Health Program; we are grateful for the long-standing support.

We wish to thank the APRU Global Health Advisory Group, a dedicated, international, multidisciplinary team of global health experts for their commitment to service.

This book would not be possible without the expertise and hard work of all of the chapter authors. Thank you for your patience and teamwork. By sharing your stories and examples of leadership, in their varied forms, you open up valuable discussion, debate, and offer practical guidance for others working in this field.

We are also indebted to our incredible student research assistants for their invaluable assistance with editing this book: Bamidele Fajinmi, Helena Galinson, Laura Hua, and Abbey Lissaman.

Finally, we are grateful to family and friends who have supported our goals of making a difference in the health and well-being of others. Thank you for your love and encouragement.

Contents

Contributors

Zainudin Mohd Ali State Health Department of Negeri Sembilan, Seremban, Negeri Sembilan, Malaysia

Sachiko Baba Biomedical Ethics and Public Policy, Department of Social Medicine, Osaka University Graduate School of Medicine, Suita, Osaka, Japan

Deepika Bahl Public Health Foundation of India, Gurgaon, India

Awang Bulgiba Department of Social and Preventive Medicine, University of Malaya, Kuala Lumpur, Malaysia

Linda Cameron Department of Psychology, University of California, Merced, CA, USA

Rosie Dobson National Institute for Health Innovation, University of Auckland, Auckland, New Zealand

Ehab S. Eshak Public Health, Department of Social Medicine, Osaka University Graduate School of Medicine, Suita, Osaka, Japan

Department of Public Health and Community Medicine, Faculty of Medicine, Minia University, Minia, Egypt

Becky Freeman School of Public Health, University of Sydney, Sydney, NSW, Australia

Farizah Hairi Department of Social and Preventive Medicine, University of Malaya, Kuala Lumpur, Malaysia

Noran Naqiah Hairi Department of Social and Preventive Medicine, University of Malaya, Kuala Lumpur, Malaysia

Nivvy Hundal University of Southern California, Los Angeles, CA, USA

Hiroyasu Iso Public Health, Department of Social Medicine, Osaka University Graduate School of Medicine, Suita, Osaka, Japan

Siti Zaharah Jamaluddin Faculty of Law, University of Malaya, Kuala Lumpur, Malaysia

Masamine Jimba Department of Community and Global Health, The University of Tokyo, Tokyo, Japan

Jae Kwan Jun National Cancer Control Institute, National Cancer Center, Goyang, Republic of Korea

Junko Kiriya Department of Community and Global Health, The University of Tokyo, Tokyo, Japan

Shubha Kumar University of Southern California, Los Angeles, CA, USA

Brendan Maher R U OK?, Sydney, NSW, Australia

Judith McCool School of Population Health, University of Auckland, Auckland, New Zealand

Salut Muhidin Macquarie University in Sydney, Sydney, NSW, Australia

Marleen Nilesse Fred Hollows Foundation NZ, Auckland, New Zealand

Sajaratulnisah Othman Department of Primary Care Medicine, University Malaya Medical Centre, Kuala Lumpur, Malaysia

Jerico F. Pardosi School of Public Health and Community Medicine, University of New South Wales (UNSW), Sydney, NSW, Australia

Devi Peramalah Department of Social and Preventive Medicine, University of Malaya, Kuala Lumpur, Malaysia

Rachmalina Prasodjo National Institute of Health Research and Development (NIHRD), The Ministry of Health-Indonesia, South Jakarta, Indonesia

Jonathan Samet Department of Epidemiology, Office of the Dean, Colorado School of Public Health, Aurora, CO, USA

Akira Shibanuma Department of Community and Global Health, The University of Tokyo, Tokyo, Japan

Luz Myriam Reynales Shigematsu National Institute of Public Health, Cuernavaca, Mexico

Biu Sikivou Pacific Eye Institute, Suva, Fiji

Maria Silalahi Community Health Division, Nusa Tengarra Timur (NTT) Provincial Health, Kota Kupang, Nusa Tenggara Timur, Indonesia

John Szetu Regional Eye Center, Honiara, Solomon Islands

Kumiko Takanashi International Life Sciences Institute Japan Center for Health Promotion, Tokyo, Japan

Jorge V. Tigno Department of Political Science, University of the Philippines–Diliman, Quezon City, Philippines

Dao To Quyen International Life Sciences Institute Japan Center for Health Promotion, Tokyo, Japan

Elaine Umali University of Auckland, Auckland, New Zealand

Robyn Whittaker National Institute for Health Innovation, University of Auckland, Auckland, New Zealand

Heather Wipfli University of Southern California, Los Angeles, CA, USA

Mellissa Withers Keck School of Medicine, USC Institute for Global Health, Los Angeles, CA, USA

Alistair Woodward Epidemiology and Biostatistics, School of Population Health, University of Auckland, Auckland, New Zealand

Keun-Young Yoo Department of Preventive Medicine, Seoul National University College of Medicine, Seoul, Republic of Korea

Armed Forces Capital Hospital, Seongnam, Republic of Korea

Choo Wan Yuen Department of Social and Preventive Medicine, University of Malaya, Kuala Lumpur, Malaysia

Raudah Mohd Yunus Department of Social and Preventive Medicine, University of Malaya, Kuala Lumpur, Malaysia

Department of Public Health, Faculty of Medicine, Sungai Buloh Campus, Universiti Teknologi Mara (UiTM), Sungai Buloh, Malaysia

Kristin Dessie Zacharias Keck School of Medicine, University of Southern California, Los Angeles, CA, USA

About the Editors

Judith McCool, PhD, MPH, is Associate Professor in the School of Population Health, Faculty of Medical and Health Sciences, University of Auckland. Since 2009 she has been actively involved in the delivery of postgraduate courses in global health for the Master of Public Health and since 2015 been the Director of the Master of Health Leadership Program and leader for Global Health Leadership stream. In 2008, Dr. McCool established the Global Health Group, a network of academics and practitioners involved in global health, with a focus on the Asia Pacific Rim region. The group has received a Vice Chancellor's Strategic Development Award and an International Research Team Development Award, reflecting the contributions of the group to development of global health at the University of Auckland. Dr. McCool's research interests include investigating the role of media, including social and digital media as health communication, commercial determinants of health (tobacco industry investments and impacts on global health), and, more recently, the potential role of mobile health initiatives for low resourced settings. She has supervised graduate students on a range of global and public health topics with a central interest in improving knowledge for translation into policy and practice. She was instrumental in establishing partnership within key agencies in the Pacific region, including the Fiji National University and The Fred Hollows Foundation to support their research capacity. Dr. McCool is a founding member of the APRU Global Health Program Advisory Group.

Mellissa Withers, PhD, MHS, is Associate Professor at the Keck School of Medicine of the University of Southern California in the Department of Preventive Medicine. She is based at the USC Institute for Global Health. She is also Director of the Global Health Program of the Association of Pacific Rim Universities, a nonprofit network of 50 leading research universities in the Pacific Rim region. This position has allowed Dr. Withers to apply her skills in leadership and management to increase awareness and visibility of the field of global health around the world. The Program promotes cooperation and leverages expertise to address health challenges in the region and serves as a catalyst for important scholarship, as well as innovative educational opportunities, in global health among APRU members. Dr. Withers received a PhD from the Department of Community Health Sciences at the University of California, Los Angeles Fielding School of Public Health with a minor in cultural anthropology. She also earned a Master's in Health Sciences from the Department of International Health at the Johns Hopkins Bloomberg School of Public Health and a BA in International Development from the University of California, Berkeley. Her primary research interests lie in community participatory research, mental health, migration, gender-based violence, and global sexual and reproductive health. She is the co-editor of the book *Global Perspectives on Sexual and Reproductive Health Across the Lifecourse* and serves on the editorial boards of six international global health journals. Dr. Withers teaches several courses for undergraduate and graduate students, including introduction to global health, global health ethics, global health leadership, and case studies in global health.

About the Authors

Zainudin Mohd Ali, MPH, has been with Ministry of Health (MOH) Malaysia for 30 years, holding various capacities, from District Health Officer to Principal Assistant Director Disease Control Division. He is currently the Director for the Negeri Sembilan State Health Department. Dr. Zainudin has worked as a temporary consultant for WHO for the LEAD_NCD Course 2013 (Saitama, Tokyo), and WHO fellow to Australia in 2003 (Hospital Performance indicators, Sydney) and in 2006 (Mental Health Promotion, Melbourne). In 2016, he represented Malaysia in the First ASEAN-CHINA Forum on Communicable Disease Control in Nanning.

Sachiko Baba, MD, PhD, an epidemiologist, is an Assistant Professor in the Division of Biomedical Ethics and Public Policy, and Vice Director at the Center for International Relations, Osaka University Graduate School of Medicine, Japan. Her research focuses on maternal and child health, ranging from fertility trend analysis, reproductive epidemiology, and social epidemiology. Dr. Baba has been involved in the education to broaden students' horizon by the very first lecture for freshmen, and global health education in undergraduate program. She also promotes student exchange for undergraduate, master, and PhD students, and international research collaborations, by finding synergies using altmetrics analyses and demonstrating "evidence-based" partnership activities.

Deepika Bahl, PhDc, works as a research consultant at Health Promotion Division of the Public Health Foundation of India. She is pursuing her Doctorate of Philosophy at the University of Delhi on "Prevalence of metabolic syndrome among adolescents and assessing the effectiveness of peer led implementation." Her work focuses on nutrition, epidemiology, and public health.

Awang Bulgiba, The first Malaysian doctor to gain a PhD in Health Informatics, Awang Bulgiba is also the first public health physician in Malaysia to hold four fellowships simultaneously (Fellow of Faculty of Public Health UK, Fellow of Public Health Medicine Malaysia, Fellow of Academy of Medicine Malaysia, Fellow of Academy of Science). He was Deputy Vice-Chancellor (Academic and

International) at the University of Malaya (UM) and crafted strategies to grow UM's academic reputation and internationalization which contributed to an extraordinary rise in UM's QS world rank from 151 in 2015 to 114 in 2018. He has also been the Deputy Vice-Chancellor (Research and Innovation) at UM and oversaw a period of impressive research growth which saw UM being firmly established as Malaysia's top research university. He sits on the editorial boards of the *Asia Pacific Journal of Public Health* and *Malaysian Orthopedic Journal* and several national and international committees. Prof. Awang Bulgiba is currently President of APACPH-KL, a Malaysian NGO dedicated to public health, and Council member for the Academy of Sciences Malaysia. He has published more than 100 peer-reviewed journal articles and is also the lead author for a book entitled *Strengthening Academic Career Pathways and Leadership Development*, a book used for the University Transformation Program in Malaysia and is currently leading the review and formulation of Malaysia's National Policy for Science, Technology and Innovation 2021–30.

Linda Cameron, PhD, is Professor of Psychology at the University of California, Merced. Her research focuses on developing health communications, mHealth programs, and other psychosocial interventions for individuals who have or are at risk for illnesses such as cancer, heart disease, and diabetes. She takes a self-regulation perspective of behavior and focuses on both theoretical and applied aspects of issues to address the parallel goals of developing theoretically based interventions and refining psychological theory. Dr. Cameron holds a BA in Experimental Psychology from the University of California, Santa Barbara, and an MS and PhD in Social Psychology from the University of Wisconsin, Madison.

Rosie Dobson, MSc, PgDipHlthPsych, PhD, is a Research Fellow and Health Psychologist working at the National Institute for Health Innovation at the University of Auckland, New Zealand. Dr. Dobson's work looks at the use of mobile technology to deliver information and support to people in their everyday lives. A background in health psychology has led her to investigate ways in which patients can be supported outside the clinic environment to increase the reach of supportive care, behavioral interventions, and psycho-education.

Ehab S. Eshak, MD, MSc, PhD, an epidemiologist, is an Associate Professor of Public Health at Osaka University Graduate School of Medicine, Japan, and Minia University Faculty of Medicine, Egypt. Dr. Eshak brings a broad range of experience as a pediatrician, researcher, and expert in public health and nutritional and social epidemiology to efforts to transform public health practice. Dr. Eshak has many international peer-reviewed publications regarding the associations between diet and chronic lifestyle-related diseases, such as diabetes, cardiovascular and cerebrovascular diseases. He is also interested in the role of social life in relation to health status.

Becky Freeman, PhD, is a Senior Research Fellow at the School of Public Health, University of Sydney. Her primary research interests include tobacco control and how online and social media influence public health. She is an established authority on the potential of the Internet to circumvent tobacco advertising bans and has pioneered research methods in tracking and analyzing online social media content. She has prepared technical reports for the World Health Organization outlining how to monitor and regulate tobacco industry advertising and interference in tobacco control policy. Dr. Freeman has also served as an advisor to the WHO expert panel on tobacco industry interference in tobacco control. She is Associate Editor of New Media for the international journal *Tobacco Control.* Prior to pursuing her research interests in Australia, Dr. Freeman worked for both government and not-for-profit organizations in Canada and New Zealand.

Farizah Hairi, DSPH, is a Public Health Specialist and Associate Professor in the Health Policy and Management discipline at the Department of Social and Preventive Medicine, Faculty of Medicine of the University of Malaya. She obtained her Doctor of Science in Public Health from the Netherlands. Her current research themes include caregiving for elderly and dengue and tobacco control initiatives. Dr. Farizah devotes her "free" time to various nonprofit and civic activities, such as Doctor2U Program and various outreach community health promotion programs. Farizah is always open to innovative and creative ideas.

Noran Naqiah Hairi, PhD, is an Associate Professor in the Social and Preventive Medicine Department at the University of Malaya. She obtained her PhD in 2011 from the School of Public Health, University of Sydney, Australia. In 2014, she received the Fellowship of the Faculty of Public Health (FPH) through distinction from the Faculty of Public Health, United Kingdom. Dr. Noran's research interest is in the epidemiology of aging. She is currently the Principle Investigator for the University of Malaya's Grand Challenge entitled "Prevent Elder Abuse and negleCt initiativE – PEACE." She is also currently the Head of Julius Centre University of Malaya (JCUM – Centre for Clinical Epidemiology and Evidence-Based Medicine).

Nivvy Hundal, is a Clinical Research Associate at Abbott, a global healthcare company. Prior to joining Abbott, Nivvy was Program Manager for the USC Institute for Global Health. In this capacity, Nivvy was lead project manager on international projects, including the eastern Africa GEOHealth Hub, a regional environmental and occupational health center funded by the NIH, coordinating a team of six university partners around research and training initiatives in the region. She also served as the project and research manager for the Institute's Workplace Wellness project funded by the American Cancer Society. In addition, Nivvy has focused on management and coordination of international partnerships, student programs, research projects, and events. She holds a Master of Public Health with an emphasis on Global Health Leadership from USC and a Bachelor of Science in Physiological Science from UCLA and is a member of the Phi Kappa Phi and the Delta Omega Honor Society.

Hiroyasu Iso, MD, PhD, MPH, is Professor of Public Health at Osaka University Faculty of Medicine and Graduate School of Medicine, President of the Japanese Society of Public Health, and WHO Scientific Adviser for Non-communicable Disease. Dr. Iso has conducted long-term cohort studies for adults and children and a randomized trial for high cardiovascular risk individuals to accelerate their referral to physicians. He has also directed the Campus Asia Project to increase research leadership in medicine and public health to contribute to reducing global health challenges. He won the 2015 Medical Award of Japan Medical Association.

Siti Zaharah Jamaluddin, PhD, is Associate Professor and a senior lecturer at the Faculty of Law at the University of Malaya. She obtained her PhD from the same institution. Dr. Siti has been involved with many research projects and has written extensively on issues such as criminal, labor, family, and elder law besides acting as a consultant for the Malaysia Child Bill.

Masamine Jimba, MD, MPH, PhD, is Professor of Community and Global Health, Graduate School of Medicine, University of Tokyo, Japan. Dr. Jimba has extensive experience in the Gaza Strip and the West Bank (1994–1996, WHO) and in rural Nepal (1996–2001, JICA). After returning to Japan in 2002, Professor Jimba has worked on health projects in Asia, Africa, and Latin America regions. He is also the President of the Asia-Pacific Consortium for Public Health and the Regional Vice President of the Northern Part of the Western Pacific, International Union for Health Promotion and Education.

Jae Kwan Jun, MD, PhD, is a cancer epidemiologist. He is Chief Scientist of National Cancer Control Institute and Adjunct Associate Professor of Graduate School of Cancer Science and Policy in the National Cancer Center of Korea. His current research interests include evaluating the effectiveness of cancer screening program, considering issues of the balance between benefits and harms of cancer screening, and developing the strategies for the National Cancer Screening Program in Korea.

Junko Kiriya, PhD, is an Assistant Professor in the Department of Community and Global Health, University of Tokyo. She obtained her PhD in Epidemiology from London School of Hygiene and Tropical Medicine (LSHTM). Her main topic during her PhD course was dissemination of research finding using online tools especially online videos. After graduating from LSHTM, she has been working on dissemination and implementation research using epidemiological study designs at the University of Tokyo.

Shubha Kumar, PhD, MPH, is Assistant Professor of Clinical Preventive Medicine and Director of the Online Master of Public Health Program at the Keck School of Medicine, University of Southern California. Her professional and research interests include management and leadership in global health and development, program planning and evaluation, health systems strengthening, and best practices in knowledge transfer and health education. Dr. Kumar has successfully led the design and oversight of several programs in healthcare, disaster relief, and education, as well as launched an international humanitarian NGO for which she was the Chief Operating Officer. Her recent projects include capacity building of healthcare NGOs and the development and strengthening of emergency medical systems in sub-Saharan Africa. She is most well-known for her expertise in impact evaluation, particularly Social Return on Investment Analysis. Dr. Kumar teaches in the USC Master of Public Health Program as well as directs the Business of Medicine curriculum for medical students. She earned her BS in Biology, and MPH and PhD in Healthcare Management and Policy from the University of California, Los Angeles.

Brendan Maher, is the CEO of R U OK?, an organization most well-known for R U OK? Day, a national day of action committed to encouraging and equipping everyone to regularly and meaningfully enquire about well-being of anyone who might be struggling with life. Since the inaugural R U OK? Day in 2009, R U OK? has become a household name. Brendan is a passionate advocate for suicide prevention and a former member of Lifeline Australia's senior leadership team, where he spent 7 years before stepping into his current role at R U OK? in 2013. Brendan leads a small, responsive, and dynamic team who are experts in community activation, social media, and integrated marketing campaigns.

Salut Muhidin, PhD, is a Senior Lecturer in Demography at the Macquarie University in Sydney, Australia. He has been involved in both research and teaching roles, especially on the study of population health and population mobility issues and its consequences in different settings such as Asia (Indonesia), West Africa (Burkina Faso and Ghana), and Australia. Dr. Muhidin's most recent work focuses on the community engagement in reducing maternal and child mortality through 2H2 system in NTT Province, Indonesia, and the evaluation of "Revolusi KIA" health program on health facility birth in the same region.

Marleen Nilesse, was appointed Program Director for The Fred Hollows Foundation New Zealand in December 2016, following 2 years in the role of Regional Program Manager for the Foundation. Before that, she worked for more than 2 years as Country Manager for the Foundation's program in Papua New Guinea. Through a capacity building in developing countries program funded by the Dutch government, Marleen worked as a technical advisor alongside a grassroots NGO which focuses on advocacy and lobby on disability rights in Papua New Guinea. After more than 2 years in this role, Marleen started working with The Fred Hollows Foundation in Papua New Guinea.

Sajaratulnisah Othman, PhD, is an Associate Professor in the Department of Primary Care Medicine, University of Malaya. She obtained her PhD from Monash University in 2008, exploring the issues of domestic violence management in Malaysian health care. She is the ASEAN representative for the WONCA Global

Family Doctor for the Special Interest Group on Family Violence. She currently chairs the Violence Intervention Committee (VIC) of the University of Malaya Medical Center and manages the Primary Care Services of the University of Malaya Medical Center. Dr. Othman conducts regular family violence workshops and leads research interpersonal violence alongside advocacy work.

Jerico F. Pardosi, BPH, MIPH, PhD, is an Associate Lecturer at the School of Public Health and Community Medicine, University of New South Wales (UNSW) in Sydney, Australia. He is also a researcher at the National Institute of Health Research and Development (NIHRD) of the Ministry of Health, Indonesia. Dr. Pardosi is the Assistant Director of Bachelor of International Public Health Program and responsible for Reproductive, Maternal and Child Health and Rural and Remote International Health courses at UNSW Sydney. Current projects include developing adolescent health integrated health intervention, reconstructing women's reproductive health rights, needs, and services in rural Alor region and postnatal danger signs in Indonesia.

Devi Peramalah, MPHc, is a research officer at the Julius Centre University of Malaya (JCUM), Department of Social and Preventive Medicine, Faculty of Medicine, University of Malaya. She graduated with a BSc in Microbiology from the University of Malaya in 2003. Devi has been overseeing JCUM's research and training activities in the public health field since 2009. Currently, she is pursuing her Master of Public Health at the Faculty of Medicine, University of Malaya.

Rachmalina Prasodjo, MScPH, is a Senior Anthropology Researcher at the National Institute of Health Research and Development (NIHRD) of the Ministry of Health, Indonesia. She was the Head of Community Health Services Subdivision at NIHRD. She has strong skills in qualitative analysis and has been involved in many research projects focused on sociobehavioral, ethnographic, and cultural determinants of health in Indonesia. Prasodjo was appointed as a survey coordinator in Indonesian School Health Survey and as a qualitative research consultant in several research projects related to health promotion and health policy.

Dao To Quyen, MSc, has worked for International Life Sciences Institute Center for Health Promotion for 2 years as the consultant for the Project SWAN. Before Ms. Quyen had worked for the National Institute of Nutrition, Vietnam, for 30 years and had various roles including the coordinator of the Project SWAN 1 and 2 as well as the Head of Food Science and Safety Department. Her areas of research interest include pharmacy, nutrition, and food science and safety. She received her pharmacist degree from Pharmacy College of Hanoi, Vietnam, and her MSc in Community Nutrition from Medical College of Hanoi, Vietnam.

Jonathan Samet, MD, MS, a pulmonary physician and epidemiologist, is Dean and Professor of Epidemiology at the Colorado School of Public Health. His research career has centered on epidemiologic research on threats to public health and using findings to support policies that protect population health. His research has addressed indoor and outdoor air pollution, smoking, radiation risks, cancer etiology and outcomes, and sleep-disordered breathing. For three decades he has authored and edited the reports of the Surgeon General on smoking and health, including serving as Senior Scientific Editor for the 50th Anniversary 2014 report. Dr. Samet is a member of the National Academy of Medicine.

Akira Shibanuma, MID, is Assistant Professor in the Department of Community and Global Health, Graduate School of Medicine, University of Tokyo, Japan. He joined the department after serving as a consultant in the field of organization and change management, official statistics system, and international development. He is a development economist and community health researcher who has conducted a variety of community-level research studies in Japan, Southeast Asia, and Africa. His research interests mainly focus on health service-seeking behaviors among people, including maternal and newborn health in Ghana, child health in Cambodia, and migrant health in Japan.

Luz Myriam Reynales Shigematsu, MD, MSc, is a physician trained in Colombia, with MSc and PhD degrees in Epidemiology from the CEPH-accredited School of Public Health in the Mexican National Institute of Public Health (INSP). Since 2005, she has been the Director of the Tobacco Research Department at the INSP, where her principal role is to generate the information that will guide changes in tobacco control policies and practice in Mexico. Mexico ratified the Framework Convention on Tobacco Control (FCTC) in 2004, and she has since directed the INSP's efforts to work with national and international institutions (i.e., the World Health Organization, the Pan American Health Organization, Bloomberg) to meet and accomplish FCTC provisions.

Biu Sikivou, MD, is an ophthalmologist and the current Director of the Pacific Eye Institute in Suva, Fiji. Dr. Biu was trained at the then Fiji School of Medicine, before undertaking specialist training in ophthalmology in the University of Melbourne. Dr. Biu worked for 25 years as an ophthalmologist in the Colonial War Memorial Hospital, Suva, before taking up the role of Lead Ophthalmologist for Diabetes Eye Care Program and later the Directorship of the Pacific Eye Institute. Dr. Biu also was inaugural Chairperson for Vision 2020 (a WHO initiative to stop preventable blindness).

Maria Silalahi, MPHM is the Head of Community Health Division at Nusa Tenggara Timur (NTT) Provincial Health Office, Indonesia. Previously, she was the Head of Health Promotion Section and the Head of Maternal Neonatal Health Section, Community Services Division at the same organization. She has been actively involved in the NTT region's health policy. As the Head of Community Health Division, she has responsible to monitor and supervise the districts in NTT Province on health programs in order to improve community health in general and to reduce maternal and neonatal mortality rates in particular.

John Szetu, MD, is a Solomon Islander, an ophthalmologist, and the current Program Medical Director at the Regional Eye Center in the Solomon Islands. He was previously the Director of the Pacific Eye Institute. Among his extensive professional contributions, Dr. Szetu was the International Agency for the Prevention of Blindness Western Pacific Region Co-Chair for the Pacific Islands Sub-Region, established Pacific Eye Care Society (PacEYES), and 5 years in Vanuatu establishing a national eye health program.

Kumiko Takanashi, PhD, is a Scientific Program Manager of International Life Sciences Institute Japan Center for Health Promotion (ILSI Japan CHP). She has worked for ILSI Japan CHP for more than 15 years, and throughout her career, she has focused on the nutrition improvements of children and women in Southeast Asia and sub-Saharan Africa. Her areas of research interest include food fortification, complementary feeding, hand and food hygiene, safe water supply, and information, education and communication (IEC) activities. She stationed in Vietnam during the period of Project SWAN1 and was responsible for project coordination, IEC activities, and evaluation. She is a registered dietitian and received her PhD in Health Sciences from the University of Tokyo, Japan.

Jorge Villamor Tigno, DPA, is Professor in the Department of Political Science at the University of the Philippines–Diliman. He has a doctorate in public administration from the National College of Public Administration and Governance (NCPAG) of the same university. His research interests are in the areas of Asian labor migration and comparative immigration policies, democratic consolidation and transitions in Southeast Asia, nongovernmental organizations and state-civil society relations in the Philippines, and electoral and political reforms in developing states.

Elaine Umali, MA, MPH, is a researcher at the University of Auckland where she has been involved in the development and evaluation of health communication interventions focusing on using mobile technologies (mHealth). Prior to moving to New Zealand, she was actively involved with development programs in the Philippines supporting the government to develop strategies and implementation plans in the areas of tuberculosis, environment, hygiene, and sanitation.

Robyn Whittaker, MBChB MPH PhD, is an Associate Professor at the National Institute for Health Innovation, University of Auckland, and Clinical Director of Innovation at the Institute for Innovation and Improvement. She co-leads the health informatics and technology research at NIHI, investigating the development and testing of health interventions using mobile communications technologies. Dr. Whittaker is a recognized expert in mHealth, consulting to the World Health Organization's global mHealth initiative, on international research collaborations, and national groups. She has led many randomized controlled trials of mHealth interventions in smoking cessation, depression prevention, diabetes self-management, and more.

Heather Wipfli, PhD, is Associate Professor at the Keck School of Medicine of USC and in the Department of International Relations at the USC Dana and David Dornsife College of Letters, Arts and Sciences. Her research focuses on global health politics and on developing innovative global health curriculum. Dr. Wipfli has published work on global tobacco control, policy diffusion, capacity building in developing countries, globalization and health, and health security while also leading a number of large multi-country researches and capacity building projects, which resulted in policy change at the local and national level as well as global policy recommendations by the World Health Organization.

Alistair Woodward, MD, a public health medicine specialist, is Head and Professor of Epidemiology and Biostatistics in the School of Population Health at the University of Auckland. His research has centered on aspects of air quality, including second hand smoke and outdoor pollutants, radiation and health, and climate and climate change. He has worked for the World Health Organization throughout the Pacific, and was on the writing team of the second, third, and fourth assessment reports of the Intergovernmental Panel on Climate Change. Dr. Woodward is coordinating lead author of the health chapter in the IPCC report, "Climate Change 2014: Impacts, Adaptation, and Vulnerability."

Keun-Young Yoo, MD, PhD, is Professor of Epidemiology at Seoul National University College of Medicine and the President of the Armed Forces Capital Hospital in Korea. He has been contributing to the newly constructed genome cohort studies (KoGES) and the Asian Cohort Consortium of "at least one million healthy people" since 2005, as well as the first genome cohort (KMCC) since 1993. Dr. Yoo led the National Cancer Control Program as the President of the National Cancer Center-Korea during 2006–2008, and was awarded with the Order of Service Merit in recognition of dedication to National Cancer Prevention in 2014. He has served the Asian Pacific Organization for Cancer Prevention as the Secretary General since 2006 and as the President since 2016.

Choo Wan Yuen, PhD, is Associate Professor in the Department of Social and Preventive Medicine and the Head of the Research Management Centre in the Faculty of Medicine, University of Malaya. She teaches biostatistics, research methodology, and epidemiology. Her research interests include elder abuse and neglect, child maltreatment, adolescent victimization, and gender-based violence. Dr. Choo has been a consultant and researcher for projects under the auspice of WHO, UNICEF, and National Population and Family Development Board. She is also a reviewer for several journals and speaker for workshops on research methodology, biostatistics, and evidence-based practice.

Raudah Mohd Yunus, DrPHc, MPH, is a doctoral candidate at the University of Malaya. Her dissertation addresses the health consequences of elder abuse and neglect (EAN) among rural older Malaysians, with a focus on mortality, sleep quality, and chronic pain. She is also involved in research into modern day slavery in South Asia which includes human trafficking and child labor. Her other areas of interest are aging, epidemiology, longitudinal study design, refugees' health, migration, and mental health. She obtained her MBBCH from Alexandria University, Egypt, and Master of Public Health (MPH) from the University of Malaya. Besides research activities, Dr. Raudah is active with social and humanitarian work nationally and internationally.

Kristin Dessie Zacharias, MPH, is Research Associate at the University of Southern California Institute for Global Health. She works closely with investigators to develop, implement, and evaluate global research and training initiatives. Currently, her work focuses on the eastern Africa GEOHealth Hub, a regional environmental and occupational health center funded by the National Institutes of Health. Research focus areas of the GEOHealth Hub include the health effects of indoor and outdoor air pollution exposure and climate change in eastern Africa. Kristin received her Master's of Public Health with an emphasis on global health leadership from University of Southern California and bachelor's in environment, economics and politics from Claremont McKenna College. Prior to joining the Institute, Kristin was a Project Manager for the Southern California Environmental Health Sciences Center at the University of Southern California.

Chapter 1
Australia's Tobacco Plain Packaging

Becky Freeman

Australia: Demographics Overview
Population: 23,232,412
Life expectancy: 82.2 years

- Male: 79.8
- Female: 84.8

GNI per capita: $42,822
Total fertility rate: 1.77 children/woman
Under-five mortality rate (per 1000 live births): 4
UN HDI: 0.939
Top three causes of death

- Ischemic heart disease
- Stroke
- Alzheimer's and other forms of dementia

Source: CIA World Factbook (2016), UNDP Human Development Programme (2016), WHO publications (2015)

Introduction

Why Is Plain Packaging Necessary?

Marlboro is the most valuable tobacco brand in the world. In May 2017, Forbes magazine ranked Marlboro as the 25th most valuable brand in the world, worth $US24.1 billion, placing it higher on the top 100 brand list than the likes of Honda, Nescafe, Pepsi, and Starbucks (Forbes, 2017). Part of what makes Marlboro such a

B. Freeman (✉)
School of Public Health, University of Sydney, Sydney, NSW, Australia
e-mail: becky.freeman@sydney.edu.au

© Springer Nature Switzerland AG 2019
M. Withers, J. McCool (eds.), *Global Health Leadership*,
https://doi.org/10.1007/978-3-319-95633-6_1

1

valuable and instantly recognizable brand is its iconic packaging featuring the bold, red chevron against a white background, with Marlboro written in a stretched-out, black font. Even non-smokers reading this description can easily visualize the Marlboro logo and package design.

But package design does more than just create memorable brand imagery, it also serves to attract new smokers and reassure smokers who may be thinking of quitting. Tobacco packaging has been designed to appeal to young people (Gendall, Hoek, Edwards, & McCool, 2012), women (Doxey & Hammond, 2011), and smokers concerned about their health (Hammond, Dockrell, Arnott, Lee, & McNeill, 2009). Tobacco packages can come in bright colors, metallic tins, and limited edition designs (Scollo, Freeman, & Greenhalgh, 2016a). The industry also varies the packaging shape, size, and opening method to positively influence brand appeal and risk perceptions and increase cigarette sales (Kotnowski & Hammond, 2013). The cigarette pack also acts as a portable advertisement, carried around and then displayed by smokers (Wakefield et al., 2013).

However, in order to ensure compliance with the WHO Framework Convention on Tobacco Control (FCTC), the 180 parties to the convention must implement comprehensive bans on tobacco advertising, including prohibitions on sponsorship. Increasingly, countries/jurisdictions also disallow tobacco to be on display at point of purchase. This means the tobacco package must shoulder the bulk of the marketing and promotional burden. The industry trade journal, Tobacco Journal International, clearly states why packaging is an essential marketing tool: "When most media advertising is illegal and even promotion at point of sale is under threat, the pack itself is the last chance saloon for tobacco company brand managers to sell their products to the smoking public" (Hedley, 2010).

Removing this last, but incredibly powerful, form of advertising strengthens and supports existing comprehensive tobacco advertising and sponsorship bans. Plain packaging must be part of a truly comprehensive approach to prohibiting all forms of tobacco marketing and promotion.

Approach to Plain Packaging in Australia

"…plain packaging of cigarettes…ha[s] never been adopted anywhere in the world. Great argument: it's never been done before, therefore you shouldn't do it. This is the poor little stupid Australia argument. We should always merely follow the lead of other countries because we're not smart enough to dream up anything good ourselves."

Ross Gittins, Australian journalist (Gittins, 2011)

Australia has long been a leader in adopting progressive tobacco control legislation (Chapman & Wakefield, 2001; Scollo, 2012). Prior to the implementation of plain packaging laws, tobacco packages sold in Australia carried graphic health warnings and were hidden from view at point of sale. Tobacco products could not be advertised or promoted in any media channel, including online, and tobacco brands were prohibited from sponsoring any events, including the high-profile

Formula 1 motorsport race held annually in Melbourne, Australia. Tobacco products were highly taxed and emotive and impactful anti-smoking mass media campaigns were being broadcast continually. Additionally, smoke-free laws banned smoking inside all public places, workplaces, licensed premises, and many outside areas such as beaches, schools, children's playgrounds, bus stops, and university campuses. In short, Australia had largely adopted the fundamental suite of tobacco control policy and program measures outlined in both the WHO Framework Convention on Tobacco Control [FCTC] (World Health Organization, 2005) and the WHO MPOWR guidelines (World Health Organization and Tobacco Free Initiative, 2017). Plain packaging can be seen as the next logical step in implementing a comprehensive approach to tobacco control, and Australia was well placed to be the first nation to take on this innovative policy.

It would be a mistake to assume that tobacco plain packaging was a new idea. The idea was first mooted and supported at the annual general meeting of the Canadian Medical Association in June 1986 (Physicians for Smoke-Free Canada, 2008). It would be another 26 years, in late 2012, before the first cigarettes sold in plain packaging appeared on the market in Australia (Scollo, Freeman, & Greenhalgh, 2016b). Throughout the 1980s and 1990s, New Zealand, Canada, Australia, the European Union, and the United Kingdom all conducted research and policy analysis in support of plain packaging (Physicians for Smoke-Free Canada, 2008). While no government during this time period adopted plain packaging, it did lay the foundation for Canada to become the first country in the world, in 2001, to require graphic health warnings on tobacco packages (Canadian Cancer Society, 2016). As of 2016, just 15 years later, 105 countries/jurisdictions required tobacco packages to be printed with graphic health warnings (Canadian Cancer Society, 2016). Plain packaging, a policy measure that had to wait 25 plus years for its time to finally come, may now spread just as rapidly.

Description of the Program

What Is Plain Packaging?

Plain packaging is somewhat of a misnomer as it conjures images of pristine white boxes with no discernible features or markings. Standardized tobacco packaging or unbranded packaging may be a more accurate description. The Guidelines for Implementation of Article 13 of the WHO FCTC (tobacco advertising, promotion, and sponsorship) describe plain packaging as: "nothing other than a brand name, a product name and/or manufacturer's name, contact details and the quantity of product in the packaging, without any logos or other features apart from health warnings, tax stamps and other government-mandated information or markings; prescribed font style and size; and standardized shape, size and materials. There should be no advertising or promotion inside or attached to the package or on individual cigarettes or other tobacco products" (World Health Organization, 2016).

In practice, this means that tobacco packages are dominated by health warnings and are devoid of any logos and other design elements. Tobacco brand names are retained on the packs but must be printed in a standard font and size. Australian plain packaging law dictates the color of the box, a drab dark brown, and that the box must be constructed of rigid cardboard only with no shiny finishes or other embellishments. See Figs. 1.1 and 1.2 for full details of the prescribed cigarette pack front and back. The legislation also standardized the appearance of cigarettes and limited them to be either plain white or plain white with an "imitation cork"

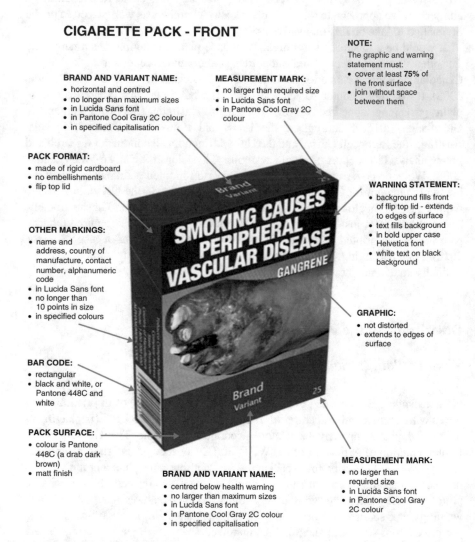

Fig. 1.1 Australian standardized tobacco plain packaging (cigarette front). Source: (Australian Government Department of Health, 2014)

CIGARETTE PACK - BACK

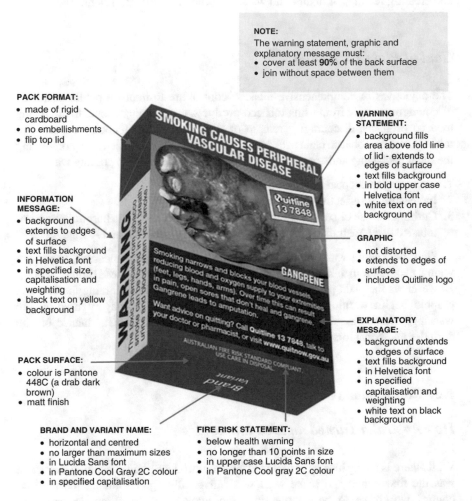

NOTE:
The warning statement, graphic and explanatory message must:
- cover at least **90%** of the back surface
- join without space between them

PACK FORMAT:
- made of rigid cardboard
- no embellishments
- flip top lid

INFORMATION MESSAGE:
- background extends to edges of surface
- text fills background
- in Helvetica font
- in specified size, capitalisation and weighting
- black text on yellow background

PACK SURFACE:
- colour is Pantone 448C (a drab dark brown)
- matt finish

WARNING STATEMENT:
- background fills area above fold line of lid - extends to edges of surface
- text fills background
- in bold upper case Helvetica font
- white text on red background

GRAPHIC
- not distorted
- extends to edges of surface
- includes Quitline logo

EXPLANATORY MESSAGE:
- background extends to edges of surface
- text fills background
- in Helvetica font
- in specified capitalisation and weighting
- white text on black background

BRAND AND VARIANT NAME:
- horizontal and centred
- no larger than maximum sizes
- in Lucida Sans font
- in Pantone Cool Gray 2C colour
- in specified capitalisation

FIRE RISK STATEMENT:
- below health warning
- no longer than 10 points in size
- in upper case Lucida Sans font
- in Pantone Cool gray 2C colour

Fig. 1.2 Australian standardized tobacco plain packaging (cigarette back). Source: (Australian Government Department of Health, 2014)

filter. Other forms of tobacco, such as roll-your-own or loose tobacco, and cigars must also be sold in plain packages.

The final agreed design of plain packages was a result of extensive consumer testing and consultation with tobacco control experts. The final drab dark brown color was chosen as consumers found: "this color to be less appealing, to contain cigarettes that were perceived to be more harmful to health, of lower quality, and to make it harder to quit smoking. Additionally, this color was not at all similar to any existing cigarette brand and failed to generate any positive associations for consumers. While a dark brown colored pack also tested well on these elements, it elicited unintended positive associations such as reminding consumers of chocolate and creating feelings of luxury and warmth."(Parr, Tan, Ell, & Miller, 2011)

Goal of Plain Packaging

The objectives of comprehensive tobacco control are to improve public health by discouraging people from using tobacco products, encouraging people to quit using tobacco products, discouraging relapse of tobacco use, and reducing exposure to tobacco smoke. Tobacco plain packaging contributes to these objectives by regulating the retail packaging and appearance of tobacco products in three primary ways:

1. Lessening the appeal of tobacco products
2. Increasing the effectiveness of health warnings
3. Curbing the use of packaging to mislead consumers about the harmful effects of tobacco use (Australian Government Department of Health and Ageing, 2012)

Plain packaging was primarily conceived as a prevention measure, to protect young people from taking up smoking (Freeman, Chapman, & Rimmer, 2008). However, as the plain packaging design also coincided with enlarging the on-pack graphic health warnings and refreshing the content and imagery used in the warnings, there was also a possibility of the policy having an influence on the attitudes and behaviors of current smokers.

Key Components of Leadership

How Australia Turned an Idea into a Law

While there is a long history of global efforts to introduce plain packaging, Australia was the first country to make what was universally agreed among the tobacco control workforce to be a good idea, an actual law. As plain packaging is recommended, although not required, under the WHO FCTC, it can be considered a standard that parties to the convention should aim to adopt. Other nations that are seeking to adopt plain packaging reforms or other innovative public health policies can draw from the many lessons and reflections gleaned from examining Australia's experience (Chapman & Freeman, 2014). Outlined below are just four of the lessons learned that lead to tobacco being sold in drab, dark brown packs emblazoned with large graphic health warnings.

1. The Irreplaceability of a Committed and Prepared Political Champion

Plain packaging would never have achieved any traction if it were not for the Australian Health Minister, Nicola Roxon, who both championed the policy and fearlessly took on the tobacco industry in defending it. It is difficult to say exactly how to cultivate such an astute and supportive political leader, but she prioritized prevention and understood that tobacco control action was essential to any preventive health agenda. She has been described as "simply the best and most courageous minister for prevention Australia has seen" (Chapman & Freeman, 2014).

Identifying politicians that understand the importance of prevention in public health and assisting them to implement policies that help them to deliver preventive health gains is a starting point. Health ministers, like all politicians, are inundated with requests for more funding for an ever-increasing list of priorities. Preventive health polices, like plain packaging, where the implementation and ongoing costs are largely borne out by external groups, in this case the tobacco industry, have the added bonus of not requiring the politician to find additional resources.

2. The Importance of a United and Organized Tobacco Control Workforce

When the established tobacco control expert Professor Simon Chapman interviewed Nicola Roxan for his in-depth book about how plain packaging reforms came to be adopted in Australia, she emphasized the effectiveness and coherence of the tobacco control workforce in Australia in convincing her it was the right thing to do (Chapman & Freeman, 2014). She elaborated that it was uncommon to encounter such a coordinated group who all "sang from the same song sheet." She further stressed that "so not 10 different people all asking for 20 different things. That happens much more rarely than you would imagine in politics. I think the value of the cut-through of a message like that, and how easy it then is for governments to pick it up, shouldn't be underestimated"(Chapman & Freeman, 2014).

The development of tobacco control coalitions and ensuring effective communication between advocates, researchers, health professionals, lawyers, public servants, politicians, and political staff is essential are securing innovative policy change. This also leads into the next key lesson of effectively countering the opposition, by first ensuring the public health side is prepared to present a united and disciplined front.

3. A Willingness to Study and Counter the Opposition

When the then Australian Prime Minister Kevin Rudd announced in April 2010 that Australia would be the first nation in the world to adopt standardized, plain packaging of tobacco products, the pushback from the tobacco industry and its allies was strong and immediate (Kelly, Maher, & AAP, 2011). The tobacco industry has a long and consistent history of objecting to, and interfering with, the adoption of policies that reduce both the demand for tobacco products and the social acceptability of smoking (Simon Chapman & Carter, 2003). On the surface, plain packaging could be seen as just the next policy in a very long line of polices that the tobacco industry railed against in an effort to maintain tobacco use and sales. However, in the years preceding the plain packaging announcement, the Australian tobacco industry had largely disappeared from directly commenting and campaigning publicly on changes in Australian tobacco control policy (Cadzow, 2008; McLeod, Wakefield, Chapman, Smith, & Durkin, 2009). The planned plain packaging laws marked a dramatic change in tobacco industry tactics and saw the industry not only appearing in news articles and programs but also launching its own paid media campaigns. For example, in August 2010 the Alliance of Australian Retailers [AAR] launched national advertisements online, in newspapers, on television, and radio featuring actor portrayals of concerned retailers saying that plain packaging would not work and would damage their businesses. Following this high-profile media campaign, an Australian investigative news program revealed the extent of tobacco industry involvement with the formation and funding of the AAR. On the day the AAR was formed, it received funds from the three main tobacco companies operating in Australia: Imperial Tobacco Australia (AUD$1 million), British American Tobacco Australia (AUD$2.2 million), and Philip Morris (AUD$2.1 million) (Scollo et al., 2016a).

The AAR campaign appeared to backfire. A survey of 2101 Australians in Victoria found that it failed to persuade people that plain packaging would not be effective, with 86.2% saying that it made no difference to their views about plain packaging. Furthermore 8.4% of respondents claimed that the advertisement actually *increased* their support for plain pack reforms (Quit Victoria, 2011).

A content analysis of online commentary reacting to the news coverage of the plain packaging announcement summarized the most common arguments against plain packaging. Over one-quarter (27.1%) of those opposed simply did not believe that plain packaging would work to reduce smoking (Freeman, 2011). Other arguments included that it was a "nanny state" policy, there were legal impediments in place that would prevent it from being implemented, people would find ways around the law, and it was that start of slippery slope that would see other goods in plain packages. See Table 1.1 for full list of opposition arguments in descending order of frequency.

A key strategy was addressing the plain packaging "won't work" argument through research evidence gathered and synthesized and then disseminated through countless news articles and interviews, opinion pieces, blog posts, and social media posts. The Cancer Council Victoria and Quit Victoria, Australian non-government agencies, prepared an electronic, comprehensive plain packaging evidence review. The review

Table 1.1 Summary of the arguments (*n* = 761) made opposing plain packaging of tobacco products

Argument	N (proportion %)
Plain packaging "won't work"	206 (27.1)
Anti-Labor Party/anti-Prime Minister Rudd	117 (15.4)
Distraction from tobacco tax increase	77 (10.1)
Nanny state policy	66 (8.7)
Other health problems more important	63 (8.3)
Legal impediments	52 (6.8)
Smoking is only about addiction	45 (5.9)
It won't stop kids smoking	45 (5.9)
People will find ways to get around the law	45 (5.9)
The tobacco industry will benefit	23 (3.0)
Slippery slope—what will be next?	22 (2.9)

Source: (Freeman, 2011)

summarized all the then available 25 published experimental studies that examined the likely impact of plain packaging on young people and current smokers (Quit Victoria and Cancer Council Victoria, 2011). The primary finding of these studies was that adults and adolescents perceive cigarettes in plain packs to be less appealing, less palatable, less satisfying, and of lower quality compared to cigarettes in current packaging. Plain packaging would also affect young people's perceptions about the characteristics and status of the people who smoke particular brands. It must also be highlighted that the degree to which the tobacco industry protested against plain packaging suggests the public health community was on to a winning policy.

It was fully expected that the tobacco industry would issue legal challenges to plain packaging laws and initial arguments opposed to plain packaging questioned whether it was indeed a "legal" policy. The Australian government was prepared for and well-resourced to take on these legal challenges. The industry launched three separate legal challenges: firstly, to the Australian domestic court (Liberman, 2013); next, through an investment treaty with Hong Kong; and finally, by supporting four countries (Cuba, Honduras, Indonesia, and the Dominic Republic) to file disputes through the World Trade Organization [WTO] (Voon & Mitchell, 2011). Two of the three disputes have been resolved, in the Australian governments favor. In May 2017, leaked documents suggested that the WTO would also rule in the government's favor, but this is not expected to be confirmed until July 2017 (ABC News, 2017). Threatening legal action, regardless of how unlikely it is that tobacco industry will be successful, is standard practice when governments move to enact innovative public health legislation (Mitchell & Voon, 2014). The tobacco industry knows that the very threat of legal action can be enough to stave off government from acting—especially governments that lack significant financial resources or access to legal expertise. In response to these legal challenge impediments, Bloomberg Philanthropies, in partnership with the Bill and Melinda Gates foundation, has established a $US4million fund to help low and middle country governments around the world in their legal battles against the tobacco industry (Boseley, 2015).

4. Prioritize Evaluation and Spread Success

Prior to Australia adopting plain packaging measures, much of the evidence in support of plain packaging came from experimental studies where smokers and potential smokers were shown mock-ups of tobacco packages that had larger health warnings and/or the removal of band elements. Research participants were then asked about their attitudes, beliefs, and likely behaviors in response to the packs. Post-implementation, there is now a significant body of work demonstrating that plain packaging amply met its three main objectives (Cancer Council Victoria, 2016). Plain packaging reduced the appeal of tobacco products among adults (Dunlop, Dobbins, Young, Perez, & Currow, 2014; Wakefield et al., 2015) and adolescents (Dunlop, Perez, Dessaix, & Currow, 2016; White, Williams, & Wakefield, 2015), increased the effectiveness of health warnings (Dunlop et al., 2014; Wakefield et al., 2015), and reduced the ability of the packaging to mislead consumers about the harmful effects of tobacco use (Maddox, Durkin, & Lovett, 2016). This body of work is a result of a nonnegotiable commitment to fund evaluation and research as an integral part of the plain packaging reforms.

Challenges and Future Steps

Since Australia first implemented plain packaging, there has been an international movement to make this policy a global standard in the fight against tobacco-related deaths. The United Kingdom and France implemented plain packaging provisions in 2016. Ireland implemented its law in May 2017 to take effect in September 2017, Hungary will do so in 2018, and New Zealand passed legislation in September 2016. At least a further dozen countries are in the process of requiring plain packaging or are formally considering doing so: Norway, Slovenia, Uruguay, Thailand, Singapore, Belgium, Romania, Turkey, Finland, Chile, South Africa, and Canada (Canadian Cancer Society, 2016). As has happened with all successful tobacco polices, momentum will no doubt continue to build, and this list will grow longer each year.

Conclusion

Tobacco plain packing is a highly successful and effective public health policy. A coordinated and strategic public health sector in partnership with lawyers, bureaucrats, and political champions saw the successful adoption of a world first policy. In the years to come, this innovative policy will become standard practice in countries committed to reducing the death toll from tobacco use.

References

ABC News. (2017). *Australia wins landmark WTO tobacco plain packaging case.* Retrieved March 14, 2018, from http://www.abc.net.au/news/2017-05-05/australia-wins-landmark-wto-tobacco-packaging-case/8498750.

Australian Government Department of Health (2014). Retrieved March 14, 2018, from www.health.gov.au/internet/main/publishing.nsf/Content/822B369C0196CB1CCA257D140082A2 2F/$File/TPP%20%20Your%20Guide%20(High%20Res).PDF.

Australian Government Department of Health and Ageing. (2012). *Introduction of tobacco plain packaging in Australia.* Retrieved March 15, 2018, from http://www.health.gov.au/internet/main/publishing.nsf/content/tobacco-plain.

Boseley, S. (2015). *Bloomberg and Gates launch legal fund to help countries fight big tobacco.* The Guardian. Philanthropy. Retrieved March 14, 2018, from https://www.theguardian.com/society/2015/mar/18/bloomberg-gates-foundation-fund-nations-legal-fight-big-tobacco-courts.

Cadzow, J. (2008). *Hi ho hi ho it's off to work we go.* NSW: Sydney Morning Herald (Good Weekend).

Canadian Cancer Society. (2016). *Cigarette package health warnings: International status report* (5th ed.). Retrieved March 10, 2018, from http://www.tobaccolabels.ca/wp/wp-content/uploads/2016/11/Cigarette-Package-Health-Warnings-International-Status-Report-English-CCS-Oct-2016.pdf.

Cancer Council Victoria. (2016). *Effects of legislation in Australia.* Retrieved March 14, 2018, from https://www.cancervic.org.au/plainfacts/browse.asp?ContainerID=effectsoflegislation.

Central Intelligence Agency (CIA). (2016). *CIA World Factbook*. Retrieved March 14, 2018, from https://www.cia.gov/library/publications/the-world-factbook/.

Chapman, S., & Carter, S. (2003). "Avoid health warnings on all tobacco products for just as long as we can": A history of Australian tobacco industry efforts to avoid, delay and dilute health warnings on cigarettes. *Tobacco Control, 12*(suppl 3), iii13–iii22.

Chapman, S., Freeman, B. (2014). *Removing the emperor's clothes: Australia and tobacco plain packaging*. Retrieved March 14, 2018, from http://purl.library.usyd.edu.au/sup/9781743323977.

Chapman, S., & Wakefield, M. (2001). Tobacco control advocacy in Australia: Reflections on 30 years of progress. *Health Education & Behavior, 28*(3), 274–289.

Doxey, J., & Hammond, D. (2011). Deadly in pink: The impact of cigarette packaging among young women. *Tobacco Control, 20*(5), 353–360. https://doi.org/10.1136/tc.2010.038315

Dunlop, S., Perez, D., Dessaix, A., Currow, D. (2016). Australia's plain tobacco packs: anticipated and actual responses among adolescents and young adults 2010–2013. *Tob Control* doi:https://doi.org/10.1136/tobaccocontrol-2016-053166.

Dunlop, S. M., Dobbins, T., Young, J. M., Perez, D., & Currow, D. C. (2014). Impact of Australia's introduction of tobacco plain packs on adult smokers' pack-related perceptions and responses: Results from a continuous tracking survey. *BMJ Open, 4*(12), e005836. https://doi.org/10.1136/bmjopen-2014-005836

Forbes. (2017). *The world's most valuable brands*. Retrieved March 15, 2018, from https://www.forbes.com/powerful-brands/list/-tab:rank.

Freeman, B. (2011). Tobacco plain packaging legislation: A content analysis of commentary posted on Australian online news. *Tobacco Control, 20*(5), 361–366. https://doi.org/10.1136/tc.2011.042986

Freeman, B., Chapman, S., & Rimmer, M. (2008). The case for the plain packaging of tobacco products. *Addiction, 103*(4), 580–590. https://doi.org/10.1111/j.1360-0443.2008.02145.x

Gendall, P., Hoek, J., Edwards, R., & McCool, J. (2012). A cross-sectional analysis of how young adults perceive tobacco brands: Implications for FCTC signatories. *BMC Public Health, 12*, 796. https://doi.org/10.1186/1471-2458-12-796

Gittins, R. (2011). *Under fire, big tobacco rolls out the poor little stupid nation argument*. Sydney Morning Herald. Business. Retrieved March 15, 2018, from http://www.smh.com.au/business/under-fire-big-tobacco-rolls-out-the-poor-little-stupid-nation-argument-20110529-1fb12.html.

Hammond, D., Dockrell, M., Arnott, D., Lee, A., & McNeill, A. (2009). Cigarette pack design and perceptions of risk among UK adults and youth. *European Journal of Public Health, 19*(6), 631–637. https://doi.org/10.1093/eurpub/ckp122

Hedley, D. (2010). Packaging, the last chance marketing saloon. *Tobacco Journal International*. Retrieved March 16, 2018, from http://www.tobaccojournal.com/Packaging_the_last_chance_marketing_saloon.49910.0.html

Kelly, J., Maher, S., AAP. (2011). *Big tobacco to fight Rudd's cigarette plain packaging plan*. The Australian. News. Retrieved March 15, 2018, from http://www.theaustralian.com.au/archive/politics/big-tobacco-to-fight-rudds-cigarette-plain-packaging-plan/news-story/edcb84582d8b4bb5d90074cce37b5a6d

Kotnowski, K., & Hammond, D. (2013). The impact of cigarette pack shape, size and opening: Evidence from tobacco company documents. *Addiction, 108*(9), 1658–1668. https://doi.org/10.1111/add.12183

Liberman, J. (2013). Plainly constitutional: The upholding of plain tobacco packaging by the high court of Australia. *American Journal of Law & Medicine, 39*(2–3), 361–381.

Maddox, R., Durkin, S., & Lovett, R. (2016). Plain packaging implementation: Perceptions of risk and prestige of cigarette brands among aboriginal and Torres Strait islander people. *Australian and New Zealand Journal of Public Health, 40*(3), 221–225.

McLeod, K., Wakefield, M., Chapman, S., Smith, K. C., & Durkin, S. (2009). Changes in the news representation of smokers and tobacco-related media advocacy from 1995 to 2005 in Australia. *Journal of Epidemiology and Community Health, 63*, 215–220.

Mitchell, A. D., & Voon, T. (Eds.). (2014). *The global tobacco epidemic and the law*. Cheltenham, UK: Edward Elgar Publishing, Limited.

Parr, V., Tan, B., Ell, P., Miller, K. (2011). *Market research to determine effective plain packaging of tobacco products*. Prepared for Department of Health and Aging. GfK Blue Moon. Retrieved March 16, 2018, from https://www.health.gov.au/internet/main/publishing.nsf/Content/C5E90158113E0DC6CA257D120011725C/$File/Market%20Research%20-%20Plain%20Packaging%20of%20Tobacco%20Products.pdf.

Physicians for Smoke-Free Canada. (2008). *The plot against plain packaging*. Retrieved March 16, 2018, from http://www.smoke-free.ca/pdf_1/plotagainstplainpackaging-apr1'.pdf.

Quit Victoria. (2011). *Tobacco industry persuades people to support plain packaging of cigarettes [Media release]*. Retrieved March 15, 2018, from http://www.quit.org.au/media/article.aspx?ContentID=27_mar_201103.

Quit Victoria, Cancer Council Victoria. (2011). *Plain packaging of cigarettes: A review of the evidence*. Retrieved March 16, 2018, from https://www.cancervic.org.au/plainfacts/browse.asp?ContainerID=plainfacts-evidence.

Scollo, M. (2012). Figure I.2. Major tobacco promotion & tobacco control policies versus regular smoking & per capita consumption of tobacco products, Australia 1910 to 1960 (5-yrly), 1960 to 2010 in Introduction. M. Scollo & M. Winstanley (Eds.), *Tobacco in Australia: Facts and issues*. Retrieved March 14, 2018, from http://www.tobaccoinaustralia.org.au/introduction.

Scollo, M., Freeman, B., & Greenhalgh, E. (2016a). 11.10 packaging as promotion. In M. Scollo & M. Winstanley (Eds.), *Tobacco in Australia: Facts and issues*. Melbourne: Cancer Council Victoria. Retrieved March 15, 2018, from http://www.tobaccoinaustralia.org.au/chapter-11-advertising/11-10-tobacco-display-as-advertising1.

Scollo, M., Freeman, B., Greenhalgh, E. (2016b). *11.10.8 Milestones in adoption of legislation. 11.10 Packaging as promotion*. Tobacco in Australia: Facts and issues. Retrieved March 16, 2018, from http://www.tobaccoinaustralia.org.au/chapter-11-advertising/11-10-tobacco-display-as-advertising1.

United Nations Development Programme (UNDP) (2016). *Human development report 2016*. Retrieved March 14, 2018, from http://hdr.undp.org/sites/default/files/2016_human_development_report.pdf.

Voon, T., & Mitchell, A. (2011). Face off: Assessing WTO challenges to Australia's scheme for plain tobacco packaging. *Pub. L. Rev., 22*, 218–236.

Wakefield, M., Coomber, K., Zacher, M., Durkin, S., Brennan, E., & Scollo, M. (2015). Australian adult smokers' responses to plain packaging with larger graphic health warnings 1 year after implementation: Results from a national cross-sectional tracking survey. *Tobacco Control, 24*(Suppl 2), ii17–ii25. https://doi.org/10.1136/tobaccocontrol-2014-052050

Wakefield, M. A., Zacher, M., Bayly, M., Brennan, E., Dono, J., & Miller, C. (2013). The silent salesman: An observational study of personal tobacco pack displays at outdoor café strips in Australia. *Tobacco Control, 23*, 339–344.

White, V., Williams, T., & Wakefield, M. (2015). Has the introduction of plain packaging with larger graphic health warnings changed adolescents' perceptions of cigarette packs and brands? *Tobacco Control, 24*(Suppl 2), ii42–ii49. https://doi.org/10.1136/tobaccocontrol-2014-052084

World Health Organization (WHO). (2005). *WHO framework convention on tobacco control*. Retrieved March 16, 2018, from http://apps.who.int/iris/bitstream/10665/42811/1/9241591013.pdf?ua=1.

World Health Organization (WHO). (2015). *WHO statistical profile*. Retrieved March 14, 2018, from http://www.who.int/countries/en/.

World Health Organization (WHO). (2016). *Plain packaging of tobacco products. Evidence, design, and implementation*. Retrieved March 16, 2018, from http://apps.who.int/iris/bitstream/10665/207478/1/9789241565226_eng.pdf?ua=1.

World Health Organization (WHO), Tobacco Free Initiative. (2017). *MPOWER brochures and other resources*. Retrieved March 10, 2018, from http://www.who.int/tobacco/mpower/publications/en/

Discussion Questions

1. What historical factors helped set the stage for tobacco plain packaging in Australia? How did international organizations and other governments support the success of this program?
2. What guidelines and recommendations are outlined in the FCTC and MPOWER?
3. What can other public health advocates learn from the plain packaging success in Australia?
4. Countering opposing arguments is a key public health advocacy strategy. How would you counter opposition for other health issues, such as gun control or sugar tax increases?
5. How can nations with less resources than countries like Australia adopt policies that are likely to be subject to costly legal challenges? How do corporations influence public policy? How can or should this be managed?

Follow-Up Readings

Chapman, S., Freeman, B. (2014). *Removing the emperor's clothes: Australia and tobacco plain packaging*. Sydney: Sydney University Press. Retrieved from: http://purl.library.usyd.edu.au/sup/9781743323977.

Maddox, R., Durkin, S., Lovett, R. (2016). Plain packaging implementation: Perceptions of risk and prestige of cigarette brands among Aboriginal and Torres Strait Islander people. *Australian and New Zealand Journal of Public Health, 40*(3):221–5.

Mitchell, A.D., Voon, T., (2014). *The global tobacco epidemic and the law*. Cheltenham, UK: Edward Elgar Publishing, Limited.

Scollo, M.M., Freeman, B., Greenhalgh, E.M. (2016). Packaging as promotion. 11.10. In Scollo, M.M. and Winstanley, M.H. (editors). Tobacco in Australia: Facts and issues. Melbourne: Cancer Council Victoria. Retrieved from: http://www.tobaccoinaustralia.org.au/chapter-11-advertising/11-10-tobacco-display-as-advertising1.

Wakefield, M.A., Zacher, M., Bayly, M., Brennan, E., Dono, J., Miller, C., et al. (2013). The silent salesman: An observational study of personal tobacco pack display at outdoor café strips in Australia. *Tobacco Control, 23*:339–44.

Chapter 2
Corporate Wellness Programs: Promoting a Healthy Workforce

Kristin Dessie Zacharias, Nivvy Hundal, Shubha Kumar,
Luz Myriam Reynales Shigematsu, Deepika Bahl, and Heather Wipfli

Mexico: Demographics Overview
Population: 124,574,795
Life expectancy: 75.9 years

- Male: 73.1
- Female: 78.8

GNI per capita: $16,383
Total fertility rate: 2.24 children/woman
Under-five mortality rate (per 1000 live births): 15
UN HDI: 0.762*Top three causes of death*

- Diabetes mellitus
- Ischemic heart disease
- Stroke

Source: CIA World Factbook (2016), UNDP Human Development Programme (2016), WHO publications (2015a, 2015b)

K. D. Zacharias
Keck School of Medicine, University of Southern California, Los Angeles, CA, USA
e-mail: dessie@usc.edu

N. Hundal · S. Kumar · H. Wipfli (✉)
University of Southern California, Los Angeles, CA, USA

L. M. R. Shigematsu
National Institute of Public Health, Cuernavaca, Mexico

D. Bahl
Public Health Foundation of India, Gurgaon, India

© Springer Nature Switzerland AG 2019
M. Withers, J. McCool (eds.), *Global Health Leadership*,
https://doi.org/10.1007/978-3-319-95633-6_2

Health in LMICs

In the last half century, low- and middle-income countries (LMICs) have experienced a transition from a higher burden of communicable diseases to non-communicable diseases (NCDs). Behavioral risk factors such as physical inactivity, poor diet, as well as tobacco and alcohol use are known physiological risk factors for NCDs such as obesity, hypertension, and high levels of glucose and fat in the blood. These risk factors are leading causes of NCDs worldwide (WHO, 2015a).

Much of this disease transition has been caused by globalization and rapid urbanization leading to major lifestyle changes around the world. Increased access to and consumption of cheap processed foods, decreases in physical activity with the creation of sedentary job markets, and increased exposure to tobacco and alcohol products have all helped to drive global risk factors for NCDs. The NCD epidemic not only adversely impacts quality of life but also inhibits economic prosperity from the individual to national level.

Introduction

Current Status of Corporate Wellness

Following the 2011 adoption of the United Nations Political Declaration on NCDs, the WHO adopted a number of NCD-related resolutions including the global action target for 2025 to reduce NCD deaths by 25% and the WHO Global NCD Action Plan (WHO, 2013). In 2015, the United Nations General Assembly adopted the Sustainable Development Goals, which recognized the negative impact of NCDs in promoting and achieving sustainable social, economic, and environmental development. (UN General Assembly, 2015). Repeatedly within these political documents, workplaces are identified as target areas within the private sector for NCD prevention and control efforts (UN General Assembly, 2012). In addition, over time chronic NCDs are expensive to treat and lead to a decrease in productivity, so corporations have realized there is a potential return on investment (ROI) in successful workplace wellness programming (Bloom et al., 2011).

Previous Workplace Health Initiatives

There has been a long history of successful interventions aimed at improving health through the workplace. Global efforts to improve worker health began early in the 1950s with the formation of the Joint International Labor Organization (ILO)/WHO Committee on Occupational Health (Burton, 2010). Early policies and programs focused largely on worker safety and health with little to no attention to the use of the workplace for health promotion. Until recently, occupational health programs and policies continued to function separately from health promotion and wellness programs (Global Wellness Institute, 2016).

Alma-Ata and Its Impacts

The earliest notion in global policy of health promotion in the workplace was in the 1978 Declaration of Alma-Ata (Burton, 2010), which stated that primary healthcare was the first level of contact with the national health system for individuals, and therefore it was important to deliver "where people live and work" (UN General Assembly, 1978). The following two major global workplace health policies included the 1981 ILO Convention 155 and the 1985 ILO Convention 161, which together required national occupational health and safety policies to support safe physical work environments as well as the delivery of occupational health services in the workplace, including surveillance programs (Burton, 2010).

A Changing Definition of Health Promotion

The 1986 Ottawa Charter was the first to introduce the modern definition of health promotion "the process of enabling people to increase control over, and to improve, their health" and included the workplace as a key setting for related programs (Burton, 2010). Nearly a decade later, the 1996 Global Strategy on Occupational Health for All reinforced prioritizing the workplace as a setting for affecting lifestyle factors that may impact worker health. A more recent notable development in global workplace health policy is the 2007 Global Plan of Action on Workers Health, which operationalized the 1996 global strategy through the development of objectives and priority areas for action including health promotion in the workplace (Burton, 2010; UN General Assembly, 1978).

The 2007 Global Action Plan also resulted in the WHO Health Workplace Framework and Model, which identifies four "avenues of influence" of the workplace on health including the physical work environment, the psychosocial work environment, personal health resources, and enterprise community involvement (Burton, 2010). The first avenue, the physical work environment, is a reflection of traditional occupational health and safety measures focusing on physical, chemical, biological, mechanical, electrical, and ergonomic hazards in the workplace. The second and third avenues address factors that more directly contribute to the growing burden of NCDs including mental health through the focus on the psychosocial work environment such as workplace culture and treatment in the workplace. Avenue three, personal health resources, directly calls for health promotion in the workplace including identifying ways to build work environments that support healthy lifestyles and eliminate barriers to adopting them (Burton, 2010).

The expansion of workplace health policies from traditional occupational health and safety to health promotion has resulted in the development of modern workplace wellness programming and has directly impacted its proliferation throughout global markets (Global Wellness Institute, 2016). While the need for implementation of traditional occupational health and safety programs persists, particularly in LMICs, existing programs provide a framework for workplace wellness (NIOSH and FIOH, 2016).

Benefits of Workplace Wellness

Globally, outcomes of workplace wellness evaluation suggest positive results. A study in 2012 of over 1300 employers in 45 countries found that the impact of wellness programs grows with the amount of time it has been implemented. Overall 50% of companies reported improvements in overall employee health after 1 year, and 80% of companies reported improvements after 5 years. After 1 year, absenteeism and presenteeism were reduced in almost 50% of companies and in almost 65% at 5 years. Engagement and morale rose in 56% of companies after 1 year and in almost 80% at 5 years. Similarly, retention and recruitment were enhanced by 54% of companies after 1 year and in more than 70% after 5 years (Buck Consultants, 2012).

In addition, current literature suggests that there is growing evidence of ROI in workplace health and wellness. In a global workplace survey, 49% of companies implementing wellness programs reported reduced healthcare costs after 1 year, and 80% of companies reported improvements after 5 years (Buck Consultants, 2012). A 2011 World Economic Forum and the Harvard School of Public Health report estimates that the economic benefit of scaling "best buy" interventions for NCDs such as smoke-free workplaces in LMICs alone could be $377 billion (Bloom et al., 2011). The 2015 Willis Health and Productivity Survey Report suggests there has been an important shift in thinking in terms of ROI more broadly than health spending alone. In the typical ROI approach, companies look to justify health and wellness programming based on reductions in health spending. However, in the shift to value-based investment (VOI), companies look to justify investment in health and wellness programming based on many factors, including employee morale, worksite productivity, employee absence, and workplace safety in addition to medical cost reductions, with the recognition that these other factors ultimately have a dollar value. Taking into account all of these factors suggests a broader, more holistic, and comprehensive approach to measuring ROI (Willis, 2015).

Program Description

Current Workplace Wellness Programming

With funding from the American Cancer Society, the University of Southern California (USC) in conjunction with the Public Health Foundation of India (PHFI) and Instituto Nacional de Salud Pública (INSP) in Mexico conducted a qualitative study to explore corporations' and stakeholders' views, attitudes, and expectations of the business sector in relation to health, wellness, and cancer prevention in the USA, India, and Mexico. Data were collected through semi-structured interviews with key informants located in Mexico and India. Results from this study can illustrate what workplace wellness programs can look like in situ and the leadership necessary for successful programming, as learned from corporate experiences in diverse global settings.

National regulation, population needs, cultural norms, corporate motivations, financial feasibility, and overall corporate culture of health can all shape wellness programming initiatives. As seen in the study results, corporate health culture in Mexico largely stems from occupational health and labor legislation, which has led to a significant intersection between medical care, the government, and the workplace. Most notably, the Mexican Institute for Social Insurance, known in Spanish as "Instituto Mexicano del Seguro Social" or "IMSS," is responsible for providing health insurance to all non-governmental salaried workers in Mexico (World Bank, 2012). IMSS also delivers preventive care programs within the workplace. However, workplace wellness programming can take many forms and can vary greatly in different places around the world. For example, in contrast to Mexico's government-led approach, in India there is no overarching program guiding workplace wellness. In India corporate culture varies greatly across companies, with the larger multinational corporations often having a more established corporate culture of health than smaller domestic companies.

Although the factors which shape wellness programming can vary immensely, priority health focus areas are often similar. In fact, physical activity, stress, and nutrition were identified worldwide as the most common health focus areas in workplace wellness (Buck Consultants, 2012). Comparable results were found in India and Mexico specifically, and key informants revealed some similarities in programming efforts.

In Mexico, the most common workplace wellness initiatives focused on tobacco control, physical activity, and nutrition. In addition to comprehensive healthcare coverage, workplace wellness initiatives often included some type of physical activity program within the workplace, an onsite nutritionist who designed healthy meals for the cafeteria, as well as designated smoke-free workplaces. Efforts also focused on communicable disease prevention with vaccination campaigns.

In India, nutrition and physical activity were also key focuses of wellness programming. Tobacco, however, was largely ignored due to the existence of established tobacco control legislation. In addition to health insurance, health education in the form of informational talks was the most common wellness initiative. Many mentioned having physical activity programs such as corporate runs or yoga and meditation classes in order to support both physical and mental health. Healthy food options that are low in sugar and salt were also implemented within the cafeterias of some companies.

Despite many commonalities between programs in Mexico and India, there were also key differences that point to the importance of adapting programs to fit local contexts. For example, workplace programs to address stress in India were tailored to include culturally relevant topics such as marriage counseling and financial

Table 2.1 Percentage of companies with health promotion offerings by region

Region	Percentage (%)
North America	76
Latin America	43
Europe	42
Africa/Middle East	33
Asia	47
Australia/New Zealand	37

Source: Buck Consultants, 2012

management courses. The need for country-specific rather than regional adaptation was also highlighted by key informants. In Mexico, employers emphasized how campaigns developed in other Latin American countries were considered foreign and were not seen as relevant to the Mexican context.

Despite growing support for workplace wellness programs, only 29% of employers worldwide have instituted health and wellness programs in the workplace and implementation rates varied by region (Table 2.1) (Buck Consultants, 2012).

The USC study found that multinational companies were far more likely to be aware of and be instructed to have robust wellness programs compared to smaller, local companies. There was a clear need for greater networking between companies so that those new to the wellness space could learn from existing programs. Additionally, measuring ROI was often seen as less of a priority, especially in India. Instead greater importance was placed on being a socially responsible company contributing to community health and development.

Challenges

The key outcomes of the USC study found there is an unmet demand for workplace wellness resources that can be used by companies in an international context. Companies in India and Mexico are already implementing a range of health-related programs, most often focused on disease management. Key informants indicated communications need to be tailored to the target population both culturally and regarding literacy or education level. There was a general lack of focus on cancer within workplace programs in both India and Mexico. A recurring challenge in both countries was the need to keep wellness programming fresh and retain employee interest and participation over time while working with limited resources. One of the most significant findings was that measuring outcomes of wellness programming was a challenge in both countries, especially in the smaller companies. Most companies are not able to track health data or evaluate results of wellness initiatives to assess the effectiveness of specific programming and provide the needed evidence base for these programs. Findings from the literature in combination with key findings from interviews suggest ROI is a key factor for motivation and implementation of corporate health and wellness programming, but that there remains a gap in data collection and measurement in this area. ROI data can provide decision-makers with evidence and information for data-driven decision-making and help to improve effectiveness and value-for-money with respect to programming in this area.

Key Components of Leadership

Successful workplace wellness programming requires a number of key components of leadership. On a global scale, multi-sectoral response is needed through collaboration between government, civil society, and the private sector for knowledge sharing, identifying best practice, resource mobilization, enactment of policies, and standards (NCD Alliance, 2016). Within corporations, support from key leadership is essential in workplace wellness programming (Mattke et al., 2013). As found in the study, top management acted as change agents in promoting a corporate culture of health in some cases. In other instances, leaders took a less visible role and pushed the wellness agenda through financial support, allocation of staff, or simply encouraging employees to participate in wellness programming. In India, some interviewees indicated that employee health and wellness is formally acknowledged as a value to their company. This view often coincided with the perceived attitudes and engagement of top management toward employee health. Some companies which do not have comprehensive wellness programing noted the need of getting top management on board to support the initiative.

In companies where leadership was not engaged in wellness, key informants indicated that individuals sometimes acted as champions of change by reaching out to civil society organizations for programming support. Such organizations often support initial engagement in wellness programming efforts which can lead to larger changes within the company. In sum, key leadership roles, both internally and externally, are essential in successful company's workplace wellness programming.

Recommendations

1. Corporations without any existing wellness initiatives should begin by identifying leadership or persons who can champion wellness, including the development and implementation of wellness programs, within the organization.
2. Corporations should consider any relevant partnerships between headquarters and local offices, other corporations, governments, public health organizations, medical centers, universities, and other relevant networks to facilitate the development and implementation of wellness programming.

3. Corporations should consider prioritizing the development and implementation of wellness initiatives in physical activity, nutrition, and stress reduction. Given that many chronic diseases can be managed or reduced by the incorporation of physical activity, healthy diet, and stress reduction, these should be the key focus areas. Other initiatives companies should consider include instituting health screenings and a smoke-free policy.
4. Corporations should understand the culture(s) in which they operate and design wellness initiatives accordingly. Employee input, cultural norms, local traditions, etc. should all be taken into account during the design of wellness programs to ensure they will be relevant, culturally sound, and actually used by employees.
5. Corporations should use existing and new communication channels as appropriate (including websites, email campaigns, text messaging, seminars, etc.) to disseminate information about health and wellness initiatives to their employees.
6. Corporations should collect data to monitor and evaluate the effectiveness and employee satisfaction of wellness initiatives, including key metrics related to changes in health status, employee morale, absenteeism, presenteeism, productivity, safety, etc. Corporations should then use this data as relevant for making improvements to programming and understanding and communicating to leadership the return on investment of wellness initiatives.
7. Corporations should reflect on how a culture of health can be integrated into daily operations and practices and use these insights to improve wellness programming and overall health and satisfaction of its workforce.

Future Directions

Workplace wellness programs are well-established in many multinational corporations and are on the rise in companies worldwide. These programs present a core strategy in combating the global rise in NCDs. The Association of Pacific Rim Universities (APRU), a network of 50 members that employ more than 360,000 individuals, recently convened and drafted the "Sydney Statement on Employee Health and Well-being." The Statement called on members to promote a culture of health, commit resources toward wellness programming, generate evaluation data, and share programming best practices with their communities. Most specifically, the Statement calls for the achievement of 100% tobacco-free campuses. The APRU Global Health Program is in the process of establishing evaluation and research tools to assist members in implementation and evaluation of such workplace wellness initiatives among its network members.

Conclusions

Workplace wellness programs have proven to be beneficial in improving employee health worldwide and represent a core strategy in combating the global rise in NCDs. Despite the challenges that companies may face in implementing them, companies can also reap a multitude of benefits, including improved employee productivity and retention, reduced employee absenteeism, and increased job satisfaction among employees.

References

Bloom, D. E., Cafiero, E. T., Jané-Llopis, E., Abrahams-Gessel, S., Bloom, L. R., & Fathima, S. (2011). *The global economic burden of noncommunicable diseases*. Geneva: World Economic Forum. Retrieved September 20, 2016, from http://www3.weforum.org/docs/WEF_Harvard_HE_GlobalEconomicBurdenNonCommunicableDiseases_2011.pdf.

Buck Consultants. (2012). *Working well: A global survey of health promotion, workplace wellness, and productivity strategies*. Atlanta: Buck Consultants. Retrieved September 20, 2016, from https://www.buckconsultants.com/portals/0/events/2012/web/wa-working-well-what-next-wellness-2012-1212.pdf.

Burton J. (2010). *WHO healthy workplace framework: background and supporting literature and practices*. World Health Organization. Retrieved January 15, 2016, from http://www.who.int/occupational_health/healthy_workplace_framework.pdf.

CIA (2016) CIA World Factbook. Retrieved from https://www.cia.gov/library/publications/the-world-factbook/.

Global Wellness Institute. (2016). *The future of wellness at work: 2016 research report*. Retrieved January 15, 2016, from http://www.globalwellnesssummit.com/images/stories/gwi/GWI_The_Future_of_Wellness_at_Work_Final.pdf.

Mattke, S., Liu, H., Caloyeras, J. P., Huang, C. Y., Van Busum, K. R., Khodyakov, D., (2013). *Workplace wellness programs study final Report*. Rand Corporation. Retrieved September 20, 2016, from http://www.nexgenhce.com/images/RAND_Wellness_Study_-_May_2013.pdf.

National Institute for Occupational Safety and Health (NIOSH) and Finnish Institute of Occupational Health (FIOH). (2016). *Improving workers' health across the globe*. Retrieved January 15, 2016, from https://www.cdc.gov/niosh/docs/2016-118/pdfs/success-stories_v01_nr04_n-compressed.pdf.

NCD Alliance. (2016). *Realizing the potential of workplaces to prevent and control NCDs*. Geneva: NCD Alliance. Retrieved September 20, 2016, from https://ncdalliance.org/sites/default/files/NCDs_%26_WorkplaceWellness_web.pdf.

UN General Assembly. (1978). *Declaration of Alma Ata, E93944*. Retrieved January 15, 2016, from http://www.euro.who.int/__data/assets/pdf_file/0009/113877/E93944.pdf.

UN General Assembly (2012). *Resolution 66/2, Political declaration of the high level meeting of the general assembly on the prevention and control of non-communicable diseases, A/RES/66/2*. Retrieved from undocs.org/A/RES/66/2.

UN General Assembly (2015). *Resolution 70/1, transforming our world: The 2030 agenda for sustainable development, A/RES/70/1*. Retrieved from undocs.org/A/RES/70/1.

United Nations Development Programme (UNDP) (2016). *Human Development Report 2016*. Retrieved from http://hdr.undp.org/sites/default/files/2016_human_development_report.pdf.

Willis. (2015). *The Willis health and productivity survey report 2015*. Willis North America Inc. Retrieved September 15, 2016, from https://www.willis.com/documents/publications/Services/ Employee_Benefits/FOCUS_2015/14562_Health_Productivity.pdf.

World Bank. (2012). *Mexico's system for social protection in health and the formal sector*. Retrieved September 20, 2016, from http://documents.worldbank.org/curated/en/706101468287156360/ pdf/767360ESW0whit000Labor0Market0final.pdfKnaul.

World Health Organization (WHO). (2012). *Global strategy on occupational health for all: The way to health at work*. Retrieved September 20, 2016, from http://www.who.int/occupational_ health/publications/globstrategy/en/index2.html.

World Health Organization (WHO). (2013). *Global action plan for the prevention and control of noncommunicable diseases*. Retrieved September 20, 2016, from http://apps.who.int/iris/bitstr eam/10665/94384/1/9789241506236_eng.pdf?ua=1.

World Health Organization (WHO). (2015a). *Noncommunicable diseases. Fact sheet*. Retrieved September 20, 2016, from http://www.who.int/mediacentre/factsheets/fs355/en/.

World Health Organization (WHO). (2015b). *WHO statistical profile*. Retrieved from http://www. who.int/countries/en/.

Discussion Questions

1. What is workplace wellness programming?
2. Who are the various stakeholders that have an interest in workplace wellness programming? What are the motivations and benefits to offering such programming for stakeholders? How might these differ between different stakeholders?
3. What are the main challenges that corporations face in offering such programming? What are some potential strategies to avoid or manage such challenges?
4. What are some ethical concerns that may arise in workplace wellness programs?
5. How can workplace wellness programming be implemented in different sectors, different contexts, and different countries?

Follow-Up Reading

WHO. (2013). *Global action plan for the prevention and control of NCDs 2013–2020*. Geneva, Switzerland. Retrieved from http://apps.who.int/iris/bitstream/10665/94384/1/9789241506236_ eng.pdf?ua=1.

NCD Alliance. (2016). *Realizing the potential of workplaces to prevent and control NCDs*. Geneva, Switzerland. Retrieved from https://ncdalliance.org/sites/default/files/NCDs_%26_ WorkplaceWellness_web.pdf.

Hymel, PA, et al. (2011). Workplace Health Protection and Promotion: A New Pathway for a Healthier—and Safer—Workforce. *Journal of Occupational and Environmental Medicine*, *53*(6), 695–702. doi: https://doi.org/10.1097/JOM.0b013e31822005d0.

Chapter 3
Growing Leadership in Eye Health in the Pacific Islands Region

John Szetu, Biu Sikivou, Marleen Nilesse, and Judith McCool

Fiji: Demographics Overview
Population: 884,887
Life expectancy: 70

- Male: 67
- Female: 73

GNI per capita: $7685
Total fertility rate: 2.6
UN HDI: 0.736
Top three causes of death:

- Ischemic heart disease
- Diabetes
- Stroke

Source: CIA World Factbook (2016), UNDP Human Development Programme (2016), WHO publications (2015)

The Pacific region is known for its beautiful islands and seascapes, diverse peoples, and a strong connectedness to faith, kin, and culture. Yet, the Pacific Islands Countries and Territories (PICTs) is home to some of the poorest countries in the world. This chapter profiles the establishment of a dedicated eye health service developed in response to the burden of preventable visual impairment and blindness.

J. Szetu
Regional Eye Center, Honiara, Solomon Islands

B. Sikivou
Pacific Eye Institute, Suva, Fiji

M. Nilesse
Fred Hollows Foundation NZ, Auckland, New Zealand

J. McCool (✉)
School of Population Health, University of Auckland, Auckland, New Zealand
e-mail: j.mccool@auckland.ac.nz

© Springer Nature Switzerland AG 2019
M. Withers, J. McCool (eds.), *Global Health Leadership*,
https://doi.org/10.1007/978-3-319-95633-6_3

The Pacific Eye Institute (PEI) in Suva, Fiji, was the first dedicated eye health clinic and training center in the region. Its leadership in eye health has transformed lives and earned international recognition.

This chapter examines how a small team of committed ophthalmologists and nurses established a regional ophthalmic training and treatment service reaching out to some of the most remote islands of the Pacific. The model of leadership that underpins the Pacific Eye Clinic reflects a clear intention to prioritize local workforce training on-site, recognizing that the viability of the service is contingent on Pacific leadership in all aspects of service delivery. Building on the success of the PEI model, a second regional eye health clinic and training center was established in Honiara, Solomon Islands, in 2015. This chapter draws from the rich experiences of building a bespoke eye health service for a region with very specific needs—from the perspective of the lead ophthalmologists. It describes key lessons learned in the process of establishing the PEI that demonstrate effective health workforce leadership at a local, country, and regional level. The conclusion reflects on the core success factors that have been pivotal to the sustained delivery of quality eye health across the Pacific region.

Introduction

Visual impairment and blindness (VI/B) are well recognized as significant contributors to poor quality of life and reduced productivity. The World Health Organization (WHO) estimated that in 2010, there were 285 million people living with visual impairment of which 39 million people are considered clinically blind. It is estimated that 80% of blindness and visual impairments are preventable and treatable. Consistent with evidence from other sensory disability research, VI/B disproportionately affect people living in low- and middle-income countries (LMIC). The WHO estimates that the prevalence of blindness at approximately 0.3% in high-income countries and is likely to be greater than 1% in LMIC. Recent analysis of Pacific outreach data suggests a change in the epidemiology of eye disease as evidenced in the changing profile of cases presented at national and outreach clinics. Lee et al. (2015) identified that the number of cases of cataract is declining (with the exception of PNG, which continues to report exceptionally high demand due to a severe lack of human resources) (Lees, McCool, & Woodward, 2015).

Access to Health Services

Eye health is seldom a priority for low- or middle-income countries, and the Pacific region has until recently been no exception. In a context of competing health priorities, visual impairments caused by eye disease or trauma are not considered life threatening and therefore are often relegated to nonessential services. Provision of affordable, accessible, appropriate, high-quality eye healthcare, including surgery to restore sight, is recognized as an implicit human right (Officer of the High Commissioner for Human Rights, 2000). The relationship between access to eye care, disability, and neglected tropical diseases (trachoma) is strengthened in the Sustainable Development Goals (SDGs) (IAPB, 2015).

Australia and New Zealand, traditional trading partners to the region, have historically contributed to the delivery of health services in the Pacific region, supplementing or remediating the workforce across the region. Eye care within PICs is delivered via national health systems and private organizations such as Fred Hollows Foundation New Zealand (FHFNZ) (Fred Hollows Foundation, 2017). Other providers have included Brien Holden Vision Institute (Brien Holden Vision Institute, 2017), Marine Reach Ministries (Marine Reach 2018), Surgical Eye Expeditions International (See International, 2017, and the Royal Australasian College of Surgeons (RACS) Pacific Islands Project (PIP) (Royal Australasian College of Surgeons, 2017). Reliance on international agencies to deliver services in-country has not been sustainable for many countries. Overreliance on foreign-trained and visiting medical teams has been a stalwart of Pacific Islands health system for decades. Some may argue the benefits, longer term, may lie with the donor rather than recipient countries as domestic governments become dependent on model characterized as donor driven, ineffective, and inappropriate (Sanders, Houghton, Dewes, McCool, & Thorne, 2015).

Program Description

The Pacific Eye Institute

Reflecting the values of founder, Professor Fred Hollows, FHFNZ was built upon an unorthodox, pragmatic approach to eye health in the Pacific Islands that emphasized the value of local training alongside service delivery; unique in that the approach is based upon a "fly in, fly out" or medical mission model which relies upon external or international expertise. Concentrating efforts on growing the local workforce has been a successful strategy for the region. Building a cadre of eye health specialists has been a priority for the small team of Pacific-based ophthalmologists, originally trained in the Pacific, with specialist training received from international institutions. The initiative to set up a specialist eye health center proved invaluable, on several fronts. The Pacific Eye Institute (PEI), housed within the main eye clinic at the main public hospital (Colonial War Memorial Hospital – CWM Hospital) in Suva, Fiji, has become the hub of eye health training in the region. The rationale for establishing the PEI in Suva was based on the proximity of the Fiji School of Medicine where a number of the graduates were formerly trained. Originally, PEI was to be established in the Solomon Islands, but due to the civil unrest in 2006, the facility was relocated to Suva. The success of this model is contingent upon the strong relationship between the hospital (Colonial War Memorial Hospital, Suva—where the clinics are located) and the Fiji National University (who confer the degrees for ophthalmology and specialist eye nurse training).

Nearly a decade later, the Regional Eye Center (REC) was established in Honiara, Solomon Islands; as from 2018 the REC will become a training facility and will share the burden of training for the region. The REC will significantly improve access to services; perform as a one-stop eye clinic that would cover all needs and reduce pressure on the hospital in Honiara. REC staff remain employees of the government (Ministry of Health) but undertake their work within the facility jointly operated by the REC and FHFNZ. This model does not remove all risk, but it provides a facility to deliver eye health services within the mainstream health system. The result is an environmentally sustainable, regional training and service delivery center. The driver to establish both PEI and the REC was clear commitment and belief in the value of a locally trained, skilled eye health workforce, with the necessary support and mentoring to respond to the growing needs in the Pacific region.

Growing Capacity in Specialist Eye Health Services in the Pacific

Building, mentoring, and sustaining a local health workforce is a pervasive challenge in many lower-income countries. Trained medics and nurses are acutely aware of the salary and support discrepancies between Pacific Islands and in Australia and New Zealand. Strategies implemented to build stronger partnerships within respective Ministries of Health across the region ensure trained eye health specialists are bonded to work in the field. The attrition rate is minimal despite examples of investment in training in other areas that has not paid off. Like elsewhere, there is little control over this issue; the pull for staff toward New Zealand or Australia, in particular, remains strong. However, the push factors can be modified. Bonding agreements are in place that ensure that graduates provide services in the region before being allowed to work in Australia or New Zealand.

Designing a workforce support model is important. A workforce may be highly trained and continue training in international settings, but the need to continue support when they are back in the country is vital. Further to their clinical training, promoting a critical analysis of the wider eye health sector is key to keeping the workforce engaged. One successful strategy is to involve doctors and nurses at the earliest stage in the process of consultation of the health sector development, for example, advocating for new roles or role recognition; this is essential to building leadership within the sector. As international NGOs are aware, presenting a case for a new position to a Minister of Health, as an outside organization is complex and often futile. It is more effective to work with local professionals, to check what their needs are and gauge timing, current mood, and climate within the health sector as a starting point for advocacy.

Building Local Pacific Expertise for Sustainable Delivery Models

The positive reputation of the Pacific Eye Health outreach team as evidenced by countries inviting the team to make return visits. Several elements contribute to this success: graduates training within PEI go on to form well-networked, technically competent teams that work seamlessly across the region. Many graduates have trained or previously worked together or have connections within their familial or professional networks. In the Pacific, social and familial connections hold currency. Although the New Zealand government (via the New Zealand Aid Programme) sometimes covers the logistic costs of the travel, this is changing, and more often, the Pacific Ministry of Health is stepping up to cover the costs of the travel. However, the economics are in favor also; outreach visits are only made if there will be at least 100 patients; an incentive for countries to invest in active promotion of eye health screening outreach. Similarly, agreements between FHFNZ and countries ensure a minimum contribution from domestic resources (e.g., national hospitals provide surgical and screening facilities and support staff). Good relationships within the eye health sector are in part due to the knowledge that Pacific staff will be providing the service for Pacific populations. For a vast, relatively poorly resourced region with a growing NCD burden, this is a success.

Developing Capacity in Specialist Eye Health Services in the Pacific

The quest for greater independence was a primary motivator for developing an eye health service responsive to the changing needs of the Pacific Islands region. This has and will continue to be a priority that demands leadership from all countries. Identifying what is best for each country requires having access to current, reliable surveillance data which helps determine workforce capacity and capabilities. Lees et al. (2015) in a review of outpatient data reported a shifting burden of diabetic retinopathy, fewer cataracts, and only few cases of trachoma (with the exception of PNG). Similarly, despite high burden of disease among women, fewer present for surgery (Lees et al., 2015). The program distinguishes and yet balances the demands of region (i.e., training and the Pacific outreach) versus national service provision thereby decreasing the reliance on the Pacific Outreach model as ophthalmologists and eye nurses return from PEI to their home countries and then are able to deliver eye care services within their own national system. For example, outreaches to Samoa and Tonga will continue while their doctors are in training, but once the ophthalmologist has returned to the country, the main purpose of the outreach team visiting is to provide that ophthalmologist with workforce support rather than to provide the services from a regional level.

This is a deliberate shift: working with other countries to provide direction and guidance while growing independence and building, from the bottom up, a highly skilled Pacific workforce. Effective, strategic networking across the Pacific alumni network has been vital to this cause. Many graduates remain connected after graduation (a benefit of training within one of only two medical schools in the Pacific), so when they are looking for new staff, or someone to mentor and train, they consult within their own network. This then has positive benefits for students, selected based on reputation. Given the relative obscurity of ophthalmology as a profession within the region, there is credibility linked to being among the "first ophthalmologist" in their countries. However, providing the right support to ensure that they are able to conduct their work effectively when recruited back in their own country, with the resources they need with the support from FHFNZ or other NGOs, has been essential.

There are good signs that the training provided by PEI and other FHFNZ programs has made a positive impact, but this has to be continually monitored and evaluated. The Workforce Support Program for graduates (nurses and doctors) further strengthens this training. This is one of the strengths in all the programs; unlike traditional medical schools, the mentors ensure that graduates are performing to standard. Underperforming graduates are followed up to determine the root of the issue. If it is due to personal problems, systems, supplies, etc., provisions are made to remedy this; if the challenges lie within the respective Ministry of Health, direct engagement with the organization is undertaken to find amicable solutions.

Local eye teams are now delivering services to their own populations, some more productive with good leadership than others. Training programs are continually being reviewed and tailored to emerging needs. For example, because of the NCD crisis, diabetes training has strengthened within PEI to meet the needs of a population in transition. In other words, there has been an increase in the training of mid-level ophthalmic personnel in early screening and hence early treatment for diabetic retinopathy.

Ongoing leadership is essential for continued development in the field of eye health. Teasing apart the key success elements of the FHFNZ model and the characteristics of leadership that has been the impetus for the program has relevance for other health sectors. Building productive partnerships within countries as well as across the Pacific Islands region has not been without some hiccups. Learning from mistakes is probably the biggest lesson. Not all risks pay off, not all systems work efficiently, despite careful planning. Other factors are often at play. In the Pacific Islands region, where relationships are paramount, building a responsive, efficient integrated health service demands the following:

- Learning from examples (in the Pacific, this has been to work alongside colleagues from New Zealand and Australia).
- Work on what will fit in within the Pacific context, with Pacific values (not values driven by funding).
- Keeping abreast with research and contemporary practice and concepts.
- Working with partners with good track records.
- Stakeholders must involve the government counterparts from the preplanning phase.

The Importance of Thinking and Acting at Scale

The importance of thinking at scale from the outset cannot be underestimated. What works in one Pacific country, with some adaptation, has potential to work in another. There are greater similarities and connections than differences: similar economies, human resource issues, finances, and politics; so the concept of training up and building local eye teams will work. For example, teams of eye health workers form local teams based in their own countries delivering eye care services in their own countries in their own setting, and this then becomes the training ground or template for other Pacific countries.

Key Components of Leadership

Competent clinicians and nurses who are organized have vision and passion and see their work in the context of a team. Building the "culture" associated with working within in a team, with a collective, shared vision and energy to see their way through the seemingly impossible to workable solutions which meet the needs of Pacific people. Leaders need to be flexible, understanding the experiences of those who are delivering services, working in other sectors, and be realist optimists. Imposing change, no matter how innovative it is without support at the base is not sustainable. This also means those who have assumed or having been given leadership roles need be fearless, confident (but able to take criticism), actively involved (not just delegating), and engaged (know the issues, open to new ideas and the concept of change). Personally, leaders in healthcare in the Pacific, like in many other contexts, need to have integrity—the capacity for self-reflexivity (own and learn from errors), transparency (communicate effectively, honestly), and accountability (to all stakeholders, but most importantly to patients and their families).

Finally, there is a generosity that is embedded in leadership that can be expressed in a willingness to provide support, share wisdom or knowledge, and offer the gift of time to provide support to others (e.g., the FHFNZ Workforce Support Program).

Conclusion

In essence, recognizing and capitalizing on the value of productive partnerships within and across the health sector is key to developing a sustainable health service. In most LMIC jurisdictions, it is simply not feasible for the efforts and resources to come solely from local capacity. Eye health has a relatively low priority; therefore, it is receiving a small slice of the national health budget. One strategy is for local government human resources and services to collaborate and partner with other stakeholders and development partners. This is especially important in the Pacific where there are willing donors and NGOs who have the finances and technical expertise to boost local efforts and then to take these efforts to a wider region.

There are good signs that the training provided by PEI and other FHFNZ programs have made a significant impact on reducing the burden of eye disease in the Pacific region. This situation needs to be continually monitored and evaluated to ensure access to quality, essential eye services is maintained. A relatively small, dedicated network of ophthalmologists and eye health nurses is key, but alone cannot make the difference. Workforce support programs further strengthens this training by building on the foundational training with mentoring a cadre of staff competent to lead and inspire others.

References

Brien Holden Vision Institute. (2017). Retrieved March 9, 2018, from https://www.brienholdenvision.org/

Central Intelligence Agency (CIA) World Fact book. (2016). Retrieved March 13, 2018, from https://www.cia.gov/library/publications/the-world-factbook/

International Agency for the Prevention of Blindness (IAPB). (2015) *Sustainable development goals (SDGs): The 2030 agenda for sustainable development: from adoption to reality.* Retrieved March 9, 2018, from https://www.un.org/pga/wp-content/uploads/sites/3/2015/08/120815_outcome-document-of-Summit-for-adoption-of-the-post-2015-development-agenda.pdf

Lees, J., McCool, J., Woodward, A. (2015) Eye health outreach services in the Pacific Islands region: an updated profile. *New Zealand Medical Journal 18*(1420)

Marine Reach Fiji: medical outreach. http://www.marinereachfiji.com/. Accessed 1 August 2018.

Officer of the High Commissioner for Human Rights (2000). *CESCR general comment No. 14: The right to the highest attainable standard of health (art. 12).* Retrieved April 10, 2018, from http://www.refworld.org/pdfid/4538838d0.pdf

Royal Australasian College of Surgeons. (2017). Retrieved March 9, 2017, from http://www.surgeons.org/

Sanders, M., Houghton, N., Dewes, O., McCool, J., Thorne, P. (2015). *Estimated prevalence of hearing loss and provision of hearing services in Pacific Island nations.* Retrieved March 13, 2018, from http://www.publish.csiro.au/hc/pdf/HC15005

Surgical Eye Expeditions International (SEE International). (2017). Retrieved March 9, 2018, from http://www.ourpromiseca.org/charity/surgical-eye-expeditions-international-see-international

The Fred Hollows Foundation New Zealand (FHFNZ). (2017). Retrieved March 13, 2018, from http://www.hollows.org/au/home

United Nations Development Programme (UNDP) (2016). *Human development report 2016.* Retrieved April 11, 2018, from http://hdr.undp.org/sites/default/files/2016_human_development_report.pdf

World Health Organization (WHO) (2015). *WHO statistical profile.* Retrieved March 13, 2018, from http://www.who.int/countries/en/

Discussion Questions

1. What are the implications of short-term international or external donor support for local or national health initiatives? Conversely, what are the benefits of longer-term initiatives?
2. When seeking funding to support the establishment of a new service in a country, or region, who are the key partners or agencies that you need to work with and why?
3. At what stage is most productive to engage with local stakeholders when developing a health service initiative funded, at least initially, by international donor funds?
4. What are the top three critical success factors that underpin most sustainably managed, cost-effective health services?
5. What resources are most important when planning the delivery of a health service in remote or outreach settings?
6. Capacity building is widely accepted as key to the long-term, sustainable program delivery. What does this mean in practice?

Follow-Up Reading

World Health Organization. (2013). Towards universal eye health: a global action plan. *Draft action plan for the prevention of avoidable blindness and visual impairment 2014–2019.* Retrieved from http://www.who.int/blindness/AP2014_19_English.pdf?ua=1.

Signes-Soler, I., Javaloy, J., Montes-Mico, R., Munoz, G., Albarran-Diego, C. (2013). Efficacy and safety of mass cataract surgery campaign in a developing country. *Optometry and Vision Science 90*(2):185–90.

Ahmed, F. et al. (2015). Can disapora led organisations play a prominent role in global surgery. *Lancet Global Health 3*(7). https://doi.org/10.1016/S2214-109X(15)00055-8.

Martiniuk, A. et al. (2012). Brain gains: a literature review of medical missions to low and middle income countries. *BMC Health Services Research 12*(134). https://doi.org/10.1186/1472-6963-12-134.

Chapter 4
Shifting Leadership for Sustainability: A Community-Based Safe Water and Nutrition (SWAN) Project in Vietnam

Kumiko Takanashi, Junko Kiriya, Dao To Quyen, Akira Shibanuma, and Masamine Jimba

> **Vietnam: Demographics Overview**
> *Population*: 96,160,163
> *Life expectancy:* 73.4 years
>
> - Male: 70.9
> - Female: 76.2
>
> *GNI per capita:* $5335
> *Total fertility rate*: 1.81 children/woman
> *Under-five mortality rate*: 24
> *UN HDI*: 0.683
> *Top three causes of death:*
>
> - Stroke
> - Ischemic heart disease
> - Chronic obstructive pulmonary disease
>
> Source: CIA World Factbook (2016), UNDP Human Development Programme (2016), WHO Publications (2015)

K. Takanashi (✉) · D. To Quyen
International Life Sciences Institute Japan Center for Health Promotion, Tokyo, Japan
e-mail: kumiko-takanashi@ilsijapan.org

J. Kiriya · A. Shibanuma · M. Jimba
Department of Community and Global Health, The University of Tokyo, Tokyo, Japan

© Springer Nature Switzerland AG 2019
M. Withers, J. McCool (eds.), *Global Health Leadership*,
https://doi.org/10.1007/978-3-319-95633-6_4

Community-based approaches have been adopted as a mechanism to improve water supply in low-resourced environments (Clark & Gundry, 2004). Community-based approaches emphasize local ownership of a public good with the rationale being that local investment will improve accountability and increase sustainable practices around operation and maintenance of piped water systems. Community-based initiatives can also be leveraged to enhance economic opportunities for communities via partnerships with the private sector enhancing the longevity of the programs (Montgomery, Bartram, & Elimelech, 2009). Sustainability, in terms of a service being available for the long term to serve community needs, is also a central goal in most community-based management of water supplies.

Goal 6 of the Sustainable Development Goals (SDGs) advocates for "universal and equitable access to safe and affordable drinking water for all." Noting that water remains an essential resource that underpins public health, strengthening the mechanisms to attain quality water supply relies, in part, on effective leadership. Leadership at local level within the community who will use the water resource is critical for building engagement and maintaining an investment in quality, accessible water supplies. This chapter provides an excellent case study of leadership development and practice in the context of the delivery of water program established in Vietnam between 2001 and 2018. Five key dimensions of the project were essential: individuals, organizations, partnerships, communities, and enabling environments (Lincklaen Arriëns & Wehn, 2013).

Background/Context

Water

Vietnam has made remarkable progress on improving access to safe drinking water and sanitation in the past two decades (1995–2015). In 2015, the coverage of access to improved water source had reached 98% while improved sanitation reached 78% in Vietnam (UNICEF, WHO, 2015). However, it is questionable whether improved water sources globally are free from microbiological contaminations (Bain et al., 2014). If contaminated, the risk of diarrhea would be high; diarrhea is known to be both a risk factor and a consequence of childhood malnutrition (WHO, UNICEF, USAID, 2015).

Government Policies

Vietnam, a lower-middle-income country in Southeast Asia, has identified safe drinking water, hygiene, and nutrition as top priorities (Rheinländer, Xuan le, Hoat, Dalsgaard, & Konradsen, 2012; World Bank, 2018). The "National Nutrition

Strategy for 2011–2020, with a vision toward 2030" stated that key underlining determinants of nutrition—safe drinking water supply, food hygiene and safety, and environmental sanitation—should be addressed in order to improve the nutritional status of the Vietnamese people (WHO, 2012). According to the Vietnamese National Target Program for Rural Water Supply and Sanitation, by 2007, government and civil society partners had constructed more than 8300 piped water supply systems accessible to approximately 40% of the rural population (Ministry of Agriculture and Rural Development, Vietnam, 2005). Despite this massive achievement, further developments were needed to enable the entire Vietnamese population access to safe, accessible water supplies.

Beyond Strategy: Access to Water at the Community Level

In the early 2000s, a number of gaps in access to safe water and adequate nutrition were identified at the community level (NIN, ILSI Japan CHP, 2004). Evidence indicated that at least one-half of the existing water treatment facilities in rural areas were not being managed sustainably in terms of maintenance of facilities (MARD, 2006). The operation and maintenance of piped water systems were sub-optimal due to lack of skills and training of the facility operators. Moreover, there was reluctance among the community to transition from ground water all to pay-for-service piped water. Consequently, the water fees collected were insufficient to operate and maintain piped water systems. Low health literacy around the importance of safe drinking water, food hygiene, and safe child-feeding practices also posed a major barrier to improving population health (NIN, ILSI Japan CHP, 2004). Although the entry point for the program was safe water, the program also covered hygiene and nutrition.

Social and Cultural Political Contexts

Vietnam hosts a predominantly hierarchical administrative structure; government directives are typically translated from central government to the provincial, district, and community levels (Laverack & Dap, 2004). These deeply ingrained systems of governance are slow to change and reflect the dominant structures of power in Vietnam. Local indigenous communities hold substantial historical ties to their communities and can also be resistant to change. Local community members who could be called upon to champion improvements in water supplies were rare. Community members perceived few advantages to the community-led and delivered water program. These factors contributed to slow progress in establishing locally governed water supplies.

Description of the Program

In 2001, the International Life Sciences Institute Japan Center for Health Promotion (ILSI Japan CHP) initiated Project SWAN (Safe Water and Nutrition) in collaboration with the National Institute of Nutrition (NIN) of the Ministry of Health in Vietnam, with an emphasis on rural areas where public water works are lacking. Project SWAN aimed to establish sustainable water supply systems and community-based nutrition models through a community participatory approach. The project featured the integration of a water technology program within an information, education, and communication program. This was distinct from previous governance arrangements where programs belonged to the water or health sectors, respectively. The main challenge for Project SWAN was to bring these two dimensions together to achieve the following aims:

1. Improve the water supply systems in order to meet government quality and quantity standards.
2. Establish effective management systems to sustain safe water supplies at the community level.

The information, education, and communication component of the program was carried out to (1) strengthen the capacity of health workers to deliver the communication activities and (2) enhance community members' knowledge and practice of safe drinking water, nutrition, hand and food hygiene, and sanitary practices at the household level. The communication activities include local mass communication (thought workshops, newsletter distribution, loudspeaker announcements, and bulletin board), interpersonal communication (flip chart communication at household visits and community meetings), and occasional communication activities (poem, quiz, and drawing contests). Both programs were designed with the expectation that community members and local authorities would both be trained and provided with education and information that could be disseminated to improve support of the initiative.

Four thematic areas of information were:

1. Water treatment process, water quality, and the role of water management union and the community members for water management
2. Clean water and environmental hygiene
3. Food safety and child care during diarrhea
4. Nutritional guideline for young children

Project SWAN has since been implemented in more than 100 communities across one city and five provinces in Vietnam to date: Hanoi, Nam Dinh, Thai Nguyen, Bac Giang, Ninh Binh, and Ha Nam. The iterative stages of establishing Project SWAN are described in Table 4.1.

Project SWAN was implemented through a collaboration between public sectors, nongovernment organizations (NGOs), academia, the private sector, and local communities as mentioned in Stage 3. Each partner brought specialized expertise and demonstrated leadership at different stages of the project (Table 4.1). For example, ILSI Japan CHP and NIN took the leadership for water quality monitoring

Table 4.1 Five stages in Project SWAN and partner agencies

Stages	External partner agencies
Stage 1: Water quality monitoring (2001) In 2001, water quality monitoring was conducted using 18 water quality parameters in 11 community-managed water treatment facilities in the Red River Delta Region for 1 year	International Life Sciences Institute Japan Center for Health Promotion (ILSI Japan CHP) National Institute of Nutrition (NIN)
Stage 2: Formative community needs survey (2004) In 2004, a formative community needs survey was conducted in 3 sites selected from the 11 sites of the water quality monitoring using 3 different methods: focus group discussions, in-depth interviews, and field observation	ILSI Japan CHP NIN
Stage 3: Project SWAN Phase 1 (2005–2008) Project SWAN1 aimed to establish a cross-sectoral (water and nutrition) workable model (described in the following section) at the community level through a participatory approach in three communities where the formative community needs survey took place. An estimated 11,000 people in Hanoi and Nam Dinh Province benefitted from the model of Project SWAN1	ILSI Japan CHP NIN Japan International Cooperation Agency (JICA) The University of Tokyo Private company
Stage 4: Project SWAN Phase 2 (2010–2013) Project SWAN2 aimed to expand the SWAN1 model to other communities by increasing the capabilities of local authorities. A two-stage training method was applied: ILSI Japan CHP and the Working Team provided technical assistance and training to the Support Teams. The Support Teams then passed the skills on to Water Management Unions including village health workers (VHWs) (Figure 1). The two-stage training was important because the training contents of the provincial level staff were based on the learnings of the first phase focusing on community level. The community level learnings were brought up to the provincial levels, then passed down to the community level through the training of the second phase by the provincial staff. Eventually, Water Management Unions implemented whole SWAN activities by themselves. An estimated 110,000 people in 16 communities in Hanoi and Nam Dinh Province benefited from Project SWAN2	ILSI Japan CHP NIN JICA The University of Tokyo Provincial governments
Stage 5: Project SWAN Phase 3 (2013 onward) Project SWAN3 aims for Vietnamese provincial governments to adopt Project SWAN methods for their water and health-related programs. It has been carried out in Nam Dinh, Thai Nguyen, and Bac Giang and was expanded into Ninh Binh and Ha Nam Provinces in 2016	ILSI Japan CHP NIN Provincial governments

Source: ILSI Japan Center for Health Promotion website

and the implementation of a formative community needs survey. During Phase 1 and 2 of the project, the leadership was shared with different sectors, for example, the Japan International Cooperation Agency (JICA) passed on their instructions of project operation to ILSI Japan CHP and then Vietnamese partners in order to build the ownership of the project. The University of Tokyo provided academic support for the projects, including the baseline assessment, focus group discussions, communication activities, and project evaluation. A private Japanese company supported the water treatment facility renovation by utilizing basic engineering technologies in small piped water systems suitable to local conditions. Most importantly, at a community level, the Water Management Unions–key groups in the communities–enhanced the development of strong leadership through the involvement of the community members. The core members of the Water Management Unions are the chair of the Communist People's Committee, village leaders, operators, leaders of health stations and village health workers, and Women's Union members. These community members were provided opportunities to demonstrate their leadership skills by organizing events such as poem, quiz, and drawing contests which helped to mobilize support of the project. Further, leadership was passed on from Water Management Unions to provincial governments, the highest administrative body in the Project SWAN2. In Phase 3 of the project, provincial governments have taken control of the project, building on the lessons from the previous projects.

Outcomes and Efficacy

In this section, the major outcomes of Project SWAN1 within one village in Hanoi are outlined. The outcomes of this project were evaluated through two separate programs. First, the impact of the technical program was measured through pre- and post-renovation water quality analyses, operation and financial data analyses, and group discussions with Water Management Unions. After the water treatment facility renovations, all water quality parameters met the Vietnamese Drinking Water Hygienic Standards. Water Management Union also improved management performance (based on pre-defined set of performance indicators).

The results of the information, education, and communication program were evaluated through a study (Takanashi et al., 2013). Caregivers of children aged between 6 months and 4 years were interviewed using a structured questionnaire. The results demonstrated showed childhood diarrhea was significantly reduced – from 21.6% at baseline to 7.6% at the first post-intervention evaluation ($p = 0.002$) and to 5.9% at the second evaluation. Among 17 food hygiene and food safety behaviors measured, 11 behaviors were improved or had been maintained at the second evaluation. Among the communication channels used in the program, this evaluation found that in-person educational training using flip charts conducted by community groups were the most effective communication channels for changing behaviors ($p = 0.02$). The other communication channels included in this statistical model were as follows: attend workshops, read newsletters, heard loudspeaker announcements, saw bulletin board, received flip chart communication, and mass media (television, radio, and newspaper). The flip chart comprised of a set of six sheets of large paper illustrating colorful images of either water, sanitation, hygiene, or nutrition topics on the front sides and corresponding narratives on the back sides. The portable materials were later used to provide water, sanitation and hygiene and nutrition education messages to community members during home visits or community meetings.

Key Components of Leadership

Enabling Factors of Leadership at Community Level in Project SWAN1

Capacity Development of Water Management Unions

Before Project SWAN, one or two operators ran each water treatment facility, and their level of knowledge on the operation and management was low because of limited training. Inappropriate maintenance of water treatment facilities degraded the equipment, a situation that was common for many years before Project SWAN started.

The project team considered it essential for Water Management Unions to hold focus group discussions in order to identify problems, needs, and to independently consider solutions. An asset-finding approach helped them identify their strengths and resources in their communities (Morgan & Ziglio, 2007). Consequently, they conceived the idea that increasing the number of members within the Union would contribute to enhancing their capacity. They then specified the responsibilities of old and new union members, who were encouraged to practice their responsibilities by village leaders. This resulted in increased solidarity. In addition, a series of training sessions specifically for members of the Water Management Union played a key role in improving members' perceptions and motivation to work (increased positivity and active engagement). Access to training increased leadership capabilities among members of the Water Management Union.

Facility Development

Well-designed water treatment facilities are crucial to the production of safe drinking water. Due to previous technical problems, the quality and quantity of water failed to meet the needs of community members for either drinking or cooking. Following water treatment facility renovations, optimal operation became possible, enabling a sufficient supply of water that is compliant with the Vietnamese Drinking Water Hygienic Standards. Therefore, both investments in Water Management Union members' skills in leadership and water treatment facility renovations, through private sector support, played a significant role in improving water quality and supply.

Involvement of Community Members in Demonstrating Leadership

Community participation played a key role in enhancing the leadership capacity of Water Management Unions. Before the project, community members had limited knowledge about water safety, hygiene, and nutrition. Due to water management inefficiencies and low water quality, communities did not trust the Water Management Unions nor the water from water treatment facilities.

42 K. Takanashi et al.

The project team invited the Water Management Union to describe the problems with the water supply and the modification plan for water treatment facilities to local community members. However, this approach was not successful in garnering support for the project as some community members were reluctant to believe the explanations offered by the Water Management Union. External government experts engaged community members to learn about the seriousness of inadequate water treatment facilities and the purpose of the SWAN project. Once community members understood the importance of the project activities, they showed more interest. This resulted in significant attitude changes and the community members themselves began to request that the operators of water treatment facilities become accountable for the quality of the water supply.

Effective communication was also key to building community participation. For example, as a result of improved communication channels, knowledge of community members about water quality increased. Community members learned about appropriate methods for measuring water quality during the course of the communication activities. They could test their own water quality and hold the operators accountable.

Enabling Factors of Leadership at the Provincial Level in Project SWAN3

Policy Establishment

Prior to the completion of Project SWAN2 in 2013, Nam Dinh Province developed a 3-year plan to expand the SWAN activities into other communities: increasing the number of projects from 10 communities in 2013 to 18 in 2014, and to 29 communities in 2015. This expansion was accomplished in part due to the role of provincial government in prioritizing the implementation of a policy on the integration of safe water supply for nutritional benefits alongside continued collaboration with the water sector in the provinces. This action prompted the provincial government to develop a medium-term plan and allocate a budget to SWAN activities. Planning, budgeting, and coordination for Project SWAN3 under the leadership of provincial governments became a reality.

Continuous External Support

In order to maintain Project SWAN3, Nam Dinh Province made effective use of external financial support. Although the province covers approximately one-half of the budget of the project, they requested ILSI Japan CHP through NIN to contribute financially to the training of the village health workers and developing flip charts—both of which were found to be key components of the previous project. Also, Nam Dinh Province made effective use of external technical support. ILSI Japan CHP and NIN have visited Nam Dinh Province sporadically to monitor the progress of the project, offer supervision, and bring fresh ideas to the project.

Formative Research: Identification of Problems and Assets

The development of the project relied on formative research to identify existing human resources and community assets, such as local organizations and materials, as well as local contextual factors, including social norms related to water use and nutrition. Previously, when asked about their water situation, local community members reported only problems. In the extensive formative research, the community was asked to identify their strengths and available resources, as well as any problems. This helped build a sense of confidence, pride, and ownership among the participating communities. Once all potential human resources, equipment and problems were identified, the project was adjusted to fill the gaps through training and materials. Through as asset-finding approach, a customized project that directly responded to local needs was realized, and the sustainability of the project was assured (Laverack, 2012).

Capacity Development and Effective Material Support

The success of the program can be largely attributed to capacity building of the local partners (Water Management Unions and Support Team) and the development of effective material support (including communications). A series of training sessions consisting of both theory- and practice-related components was organized for the local partners to provide necessary knowledge and skills of implementing SWAN activities. As a result, the local partners recognized the benefit of the project and gained confidence in the information they would provide to community members. Fostering local leadership resulted in an increase in community members' willingness to participate in the project (Kim, Kim, Sychareun, & Kang, 2016).

Effective communication was vital. Using multiple communication channels and materials to encourage behavioral change among the community members proved successful. External partners held extensive discussions on the technology and knowledge that should be introduced to communities to respond to local contexts. Health messages were modified based on community members' points of view, and graphical images were used to help members with low literacy understand health messages. Project SWAN's implementation manuals were created to demonstrate what had been carried out in the target communities and were used to encourage neighboring areas to participate in the project.

Financial Stability

The ultimate objective of the water supply program is community payment for water, which will be reinvested into the maintenance of piped water systems for the delivery of clean, safe water. Financial stability for the program was achieved by the following four steps: (1) infrastructure improvements increased the quality and quantity of water at treatment facilities, and the water supply coverage improved, (2) communication activities encouraged community members appreciation of the complex water treatment process and the health benefits of safe drinking water, and (3) community members accepting the increased water fees, and (4) Water Management Unions established sound water fee collection systems and carried out measures against water loss and theft. An increase in the revenue of Water Management Unions strengthened the overall financial independence of the program.

Future Directions

Strong leadership provides a foundation to achieve greater success for projects and amplifies health gains. Several key elements contributed to growing a sustainable water program in Vietnam: building capacity development with the Water Management Unions, infrastructure development, involvement of community members, policy establishment, and continuous external support. The supportive environment that Project SWAN created also contributed indirectly to the demonstration of leadership and consequently contributed to its success. Ensuring sustainability is primary goal for community-based programs. Project SWAN achieved this outcome by building leadership through active participation across the multisector local partners. Water, as the basis of all life, has been improved through cooperative effort to carry out the vision for a sustainable system to benefit all.

References

Bain, R., Cronk, R., Hossain, R., Bonjour, S., Onda, K., & Wright, J. (2014). Global assessment of exposure to faecal contamination through drinking water based on a systematic review. *Tropical Medicine & International Health, 19*(8), 917–927.
Central Intelligence Agenct (CIA) (2016). *CIA World Factbook*. Retrieved March 14, 2018, from https://www.cia.gov/library/publications/the-world-factbook/
Clark, R., & Gundry, S. W. (2004). The prominence of health in donor policy for water supply and sanitation: A review. *Journal of Water and Health, 2*(3), 157–169.
International Life Sciences Institute (ILSI) Japan website. (n.d.). *Centre for Health Promotion (CHP) – Project SWAN*. Retrieved April 2, 2018, from http://www.ilsijapan.org/English/ILSIJapan/COM/CHP_SWAN.php

Kim, J., Kim, J. H., Sychareun, V., & Kang, M. (2016). Recovering disrupted social capital: Insights from Lao PDR rural villagers' perceptions of local leadership. *BMC Public Health, 16*(1), 1189.

Laverack, G. (2012). Where are the champions of global health promotion? *Global Health Promotion, 19*(2), 63–65.

Laverack, G., & Dap, H. (2004). Transforming information, education and communication in Vietnam. *Health Education, 103*(6), 363–369.

Lincklaen Arriëns, W., & Wehn, U. (2013). Exploring water leadership. *Water Policy, 15*, 15–41.

Ministry of Agriculture and Rural Development, Vietnam. (2005). *National target program for rural water supply and sanitation (2006–2010) (NTPII)*. Hanoi. Retrieved April 2, 2018, from https://ja.scribd.com/document/58959260/National-Target-Program-for-Rural-Water-Supply-and-Sanitation-2006-2010

Ministry of Agriculture and Rural Development, Vietnam. (2006). *National target program for rural water supply and sanitation (2006–2010) (NTPII)*. Hanoi. Retrieved March 17, 2018, from http://documents.worldbank.org/curated/en/888701468329935238/pdf/676660PGID0VN0rural0water0supply.pdf/

Montgomery, M. A., Bartram, J., & Elimelech, M. (2009). Increasing functional sustainability of water and sanitation supplies in rural sub-Saharan Africa. *Environmental Engineering Science, 26*(5), 1017–1023.

Morgan, A., & Ziglio, E. (2007). Revitalising the evidence base for public health: An assets model. *Promotion & Education*, (Suppl 2), 17–22.

National Institute of Nutrition (NIN), Vietnam and ILSI Japan CHP. (2004). *Needs of communities for improving safe water supply and health*. Hanoi. Retrieved March 17, 2018, from https://extranet.who.int/nutrition/gina/en/node/11519

Rheinländer, T., Xuan le, T. T., Hoat, L. N., Dalsgaard, A., & Konradsen, F. (2012). Hygiene and sanitation promotion strategies among ethnic minority communities in northern Vietnam: A stakeholder analysis. *Health Policy and Planning, 27*(7), 600–612.

Takanashi, K., Quyen, D. T., Hoa, N. T. L., Khan, N. C., Yasuoka, J., & Jimba, M. (2013). Long-term impact of community-based information, education and communication activities on food hygiene and food safety behaviors in Vietnam: A longitudinal study. *PLoS One, 8*(8), e70654.

UNICEF and the World Health Organization. (2015*). Progress on sanitation and drinking water – 2015 update and MDG assessment. UNICEF and World Health Organization*. Retrieved March 17, 2018, from http://files.unicef.org/publications/files/Progress_on_Sanitation_and_Drinking_Water_2015_Update_.pdf

United Nations Development Programme (UNDP). (2016). *Human development report 2016*. Retrieved March 14, 2018, from http://hdr.undp.org/sites/default/files/2016_human_development_report.pdf

World Bank. (2018). *Country and lending groups*. Retrieved March 17, 2018, from https://datahelpdesk.worldbank.org/knowledgebase/articles/906519-world-bank-country-and-lending-groups

World Health Organization (WHO). (2012). *Global Database on the Implementation of Nutrition Action (GINA). Policy – National Nutrition Strategy for 2011–2020, with a Vision towards 2030*. Retrieved March 17, 2018, from https://extranet.who.int/nutrition/gina/en/node/11519

World Health Organization (WHO) (2015). *WHO statistical profile*. Retrieved March 14, 2018, from http://www.who.int/countries/en/

World Health Organization, UNICEF and USAID. (2015). *Improving nutrition outcomes with better water, sanitation and hygiene: Practical solutions for policies and programmes*. World Health Organization. Retrieved March 17, 2018, from http://www.who.int/water_sanitation_health/publications/washandnutrition/en/

Discussion Questions

1. What factors led to the recognition of the need to change and improve water supplies in Vietnam?
2. Which of the range of the organization involved in the Project SWAN were instrumental in initiating the process of change?
3. How were improvements in water quality measured? Were these measures effective in ensuring quality supply of water?
4. What factors threaten the supply of quality water in low-resourced environments?
5. Why is health literacy so important to ensuring a sustainable system to supply quality water in Vietnam?
6. What are the core leadership strengths of this project? How was leadership demonstrated within the SWAN program?

Follow-Up Readings

Project SWAN (Safe Water and Nutrition). Retrieved from http://ilsi.org/project-swan-case-study/.
World Health Organization (WHO). (2017). *Guidelines for drinking-water quality*. Geneva. Retrieved from http://www.who.int/water_sanitation_health/publications/drinking-water-quality-guidelines-4-including-1st-addendum/en/

Chapter 5
Successful Reduction of Blood Pressure and Stroke Risk in Japan

Sachiko Baba, Ehab S. Eshak, and Hiroyasu Iso

Japan: Demographics Overview
Population: 126,451,398
Life expectancy: 85 years

- Male: 81.7
- Female: 88.5

GNI per capita: $37,268
Total fertility rate: 1.41 children/woman
Under-five mortality rate (per 1000 live births): 3
UN HDI: 0.903*Top three causes of death*

- Lower respiratory infections
- Stroke
- Ischemic heart disease

Source: CIA World Factbook (2016), UNDP Human Development Programme (2016), WHO publications (2015)

S. Baba
Biomedical Ethics and Public Policy, Department of Social Medicine, Osaka University Graduate School of Medicine, Suita, Osaka, Japan

E. S. Eshak
Public Health, Department of Social Medicine, Osaka University Graduate School of Medicine, Suita, Osaka, Japan

Department of Public Health and Community Medicine, Faculty of Medicine, Minia University, Minia, Egypt

H. Iso (✉)
Public Health, Department of Social Medicine, Osaka University Graduate School of Medicine, Suita, Osaka, Japan
e-mail: iso@pbhel.med.osaka-u.ac.jp

© Springer Nature Switzerland AG 2019
M. Withers, J. McCool (eds.), *Global Health Leadership*,
https://doi.org/10.1007/978-3-319-95633-6_5

Cerebrovascular disease (stroke) is a common noncommunicable disease and the second highest leading cause of death worldwide. Since hypertension is the strongest risk factor for stroke, the prevention of hypertension and the control of blood pressure are critical elements to prevent stroke. In 1963, an integrated stroke prevention program was launched in a Japanese community of Ikawa town, in Akita Prefecture. The final version of the program includes five core elements: (1) systematic blood pressure screening for detection of hypertensive individuals through an annual health checkup of residents aged ≥30 or 40 years; (2) referral of high-risk individuals to local clinics for antihypertensive medication; (3) health education for people with hypertension detected at blood pressure screening via workshops by physicians, public health nurses, and nutritionists and home visits by public health nurses; (4) involvement of heath volunteers; and (5) community-wide media health education. The most successful elements of this community-based program were the regular health checkups and targeted health promotion campaigns on healthy lifestyles by the multidisciplinary health professionals including physicians, public health nurses, nutritionists, clerical workers, and researchers. The program was later endorsed by WHO as suitable for middle-income countries where the stroke burden is increasing.

Introduction

Cerebrovascular disease (stroke) is a major noncommunicable disease and the second highest leading cause of death worldwide (WHO, 2017). Since hypertension is the strongest universal risk factor for stroke (Whelton et al., 2017), the reduction of hypertension and the control of blood pressure are critical elements to prevent stroke. Japan has experienced some of the highest hypertension rates globally. The World Health Organization's latest available data (from 2008) indicate that more than one-quarter (26.7%) of the adult population in Japan suffers from raised blood pressure (WHO, 2014). Although the incidence and mortality from stroke have decreased significantly in Japan over the past 40 years (Liu, Ikeda, & Yamori, 2001; Sarti, Rastenyte, Cepaitis, & Tuomilehto, 2000), stroke remains the second-leading cause of death in Japan, contributing to about 10% of all deaths (WHO, 2015).

Background on the Program

Serendipitous meetings are often the starting points for productive public health ventures. In 1963, two years after the initiation of universal health coverage in Japan, Dr. Komachi, who is an Emeritus Professor of Tsukuba University and worked for the Osaka Medical Center for Cancer and Cardiovascular Disease at that time, met with the director of the Public Health Institute of Akita Prefecture at a conference of public health held in Osaka. This encounter and a follow-up meeting, which also included the mayor and the director of the public health center in Ikawa town, Akita Prefecture, identified a set of shared concerns regarding the high prevalence of stroke in the community. A request for assistance in implementing a preventive strategy was made and put into practice in the same year, signaling the start of a successful, sustainable stroke prevention initiative in Japan. The components of this prevention program are presented below.

Program Components

The original program (1963–1966) began by implementing a blood pressure screening program for all the residents aged 30 years and over residing in the target community. Each person screened also received a urine analysis for proteinuria and urinary sugar, electrocardiogram examination, fundus examination, and blood test (serum total cholesterol, triglyceride, and total protein), along with a clinical examination. Consultations including physical examinations were also performed on the spot for those who were at elevated risk of stroke. The participation rate in the screening program during 1963–1966 was 86.6% (2690/3098) (Komachi, 2007). Moreover, Dr. Komachi and his research team (hereafter referred to as "the team") worked continuously to undertake regular blood pressure monitoring and education workshops in addition to the annual health checkup for high-risk residents and those of the age of 30 years. The team promptly published the progress report of the comprehensive screening program, and it was later published and distributed among participants and the relevant institutes in 1967.

Accompanied Program

Akita Prefecture located in the Northeastern part of Japan historically reported the highest stroke mortality rate in Japan. In fact, it had the highest stroke mortality rate in the world at that time (Yuzuki, 1958). Even though Akita Prefecture, at present, reported lower rates than that in high-income economies, it is significantly higher than that for Japan; age-adjusted mortality rate for 100,000 was 31.1 in Akita in 2015, 64.7 in high-income economies in 2016, and 25.1 in Japan in 2015 (World Health Organization, 2017; Nomura et al., 2017). The cultural determinants for stroke risk in Akita community included agriculture-dependent industrial structures, manual labor associated with agricultural production, local diets, and customs common to the Northeastern part of Japan but distinct from those in other Japanese areas. The team began investigating the lifestyle and dietary patterns of Akita residents via unofficial reports collected by farmers, including personal household financial records, children's diaries, and history books accompanied with the health screening described above. As a characteristic of Japanese culture, personal household financial records and children's diaries were usually recorded and kept in the traditional storehouse of the family, where home-cooked, salt-preserved products were stored. Those documents were kindly lent to the investigators who visited the family for this study (Ozawa, 1968). The investigation revealed a high intake of rice and salt but a low intake of animal protein in this rural community whose residents were primarily manual laborers who cultivated rice (Shimamoto et al., 1989).

Funding

At the beginning of the initiative, there was little confidence within the Ministry of Health and Welfare that stroke could be prevented via community-based activities. Accordingly, funding the program proved to be a major challenge, and internal funds from the team leader were used to kick-start the program. A team member, who later assumed the position of medical officer within the Ministry of Health, developed skills in health financing and budget decision-making, skills that proved instrumental in persuading colleagues in the Ministry of Health to fund the program.

Results

The preliminary results of the program at Ikawa town showed success; there was a substantial decline in the prevalence of severe hypertension and a decline in stroke incidence in the 1960s (Shimamoto et al., 1994). The community-based program was positively evaluated by local residents, local medical and health professionals, and the government. In 1969 the Ministry of Health provided additional funding to expand stroke prevention activities in six prefectures, which supported investing in population screening (including blood pressure and urine analysis). The program included five core elements (Iso et al., 1998):

1. Systematic blood pressure screening for detection of hypertensive individuals through annual health checkups of residents aged ≥30 or 40 years (depending upon location).
2. Referral of high-risk individuals to local clinics for antihypertensive medication.
3. Health education for people with hypertension detected at blood pressure screening via workshops by physicians, public health nurses, and nutritionists and home visits by public health nurses.
4. Involvement of heath volunteers.
5. Community-wide media health education.

The program, in particular the regular health checkups and targeted health promotion campaigns on healthy lifestyle, contributed to a substantial decline in blood pressure levels and over a half risk reduction of stroke incidence.

The cost of the intervention program for hypertension detection including expenses for personnel, health promotion, and health checkups was calculated. The cost of medical treatment for hypertension/stroke patients was also estimated in a control community as the actual number of hypertension and stroke events within the community, multiplied by the average hypertension/stroke treatment cost under national health insurance. The sum of these costs was lower in the intervention program community than that in the control community. Thus, the program was found to be cost-saving more than 13 years after its initiation (Yamagishi et al., 2012). Finally, in 1982, an act for health and welfare for the aged was implemented to cover nationwide blood pressure screening for hypertension, blood and urinary tests, electrocardiogram, and fundoscopy examination for detection of high-risk individuals for cardiovascular diseases and cancer for all residents aged 40 years and older. A large cohort study based in Southeastern Japan supported the importance of hypertension management for the reduced stroke incidence and mortality (Kubo et al., 2003). The World Health Organization endorsed the program (World Health Organization, 2013) as suitable for most middle-income countries where stroke burden is increasing (World Health Organization, 2017).

A declining trend in stroke mortality had begun nationally in 1965–1970, which was attributed to efforts to control risk factors (e.g., treatment for hypertension, a reduction in salt intake, and a reduction of cigarette smoking). In addition, improved treatment for stroke helped to reduce case fatality rates and to increase survival (Liu et al., 2001; Ueshima, 2007).

Key Components of Leadership

The Akita Program became a model for stroke prevention nationally and provided several important lessons in leadership, which can be divided into five elements (Heifetz and Linsky, 2002). First, partnership was key. A steering committee was organized for the program with members from diverse sectors. Numerous partners became involved in the program, including the Osaka Medical Center for Cancer and Cardiovascular Disease, the Akita Research Institute of Public Health, the local public health center, and local Ikawa medical clinics. Among the key features of the program was the multidisciplinary health professional model, which included physicians, public health nurses, nutritionists, local government officials, and researchers. This collaboration enabled discussion from broad perspectives and yielded propositions such as monthly education workshops for residents to be conducted by public health nurses and midwives. This investment from allied health professionals reduced the burden on local physicians and was a successful element of the program because of the nurses' experience and familiarity with the communities.

The second critical element in the success of the program was that community leaders in Akita took responsibility for their contribution to the stroke burden and initiative. They did not push the community to implement the targeted lifestyle modifications using punitive measures. Instead, they approached the problem with a collaborative attitude and demonstrated to residents the desire to face the problem together. They aimed to overcome any barriers through direct engagement with the community through community-based initiatives. Community leaders served as role models to others through their continuous presence in the community. They made changes to their own nutrition and participated in the annual health checkups for blood pressure screening and monitoring. Through modeling desired behaviors, their leadership was important in inspiring others to make the targeted changes.

Third, understanding the contextual factors that were barriers to participating in the program activities was crucial. Allowing for flexibility and adaptation of lessons learned also contributed to the success of the program. For example, some middle-aged farmers took up supplementary work over winter in the cities: a factor that contributed to their lack of willingness to participate in the health checkups. The checkup period was later shifted to the spring time when almost all eligible residents resided in the village. In addition, the program allowed flexibility; public health nurses engaged middle-aged populations by making early morning or evening home visits after work; visits in rainy days when daily manual labor workers, including farmers, stay at home; or even targeting farmers at the tax offices during the period when they were required to file taxes. Attitudes toward hypertension were also a barrier; patients were not willing to visit clinic regularly because they were afraid that people thought that they just wanted to escape from working. However, once the importance of the regular monitoring of blood pressure was promoted, not only people with hypertension but also their family members participated in the health education workshops.

Fourth, cultural competency is another element of this successful intervention. The interventions of reducing salt intake, taking at least a monthly day off from work for rest (farmers have tended to take no rests even for Saturdays or Sundays), doing blood pressure screening, and treatment options were found to be acceptable to community members. This "simple" approach increased the likelihood of community motivation. Important changes were also made to long-standing cultural traditions by residents, and it was important to commend them for their efforts in modifying dietary habits. Traditional meals relied heavily on rice with home-cooked salted preserved products, salted dried fish, and foods boiled in soy sauce and miso (soybean paste) soup. However, residents voluntarily adopted better diets. Also, at that time, salt was frequently used to preserve foods at room temperature. However, due to the introduction of refrigerators and freezers in the 1970s, the conventional process of preserving food products with salt was reduced.

The fifth element was community ownership of the program. At the beginning, the educational workshops and the health checkups were carried out by the research team. However, over time, community leaders and volunteers have become motivated to join the workshops, some even taking ownership in managing the workshops. In addition, community leaders and health volunteers, who were also program recipients because they lived in the same town, assisted with registration, guidance, and identification of the participants. While this may not have been the most efficient approach, because each time volunteer members are changed, newer volunteers needed to be trained on the procedures of this program, it resulted in a broader understanding of this project by the whole community. It was important in making the residents feel that this project belonged to them and they became more invested in the success of the program.

Future Challenges

The great success of the prevention program for stroke was based on controlling blood pressure levels (Liu et al., 2001). However, new threats may emerge that could potentially increase stroke and ischemic heart disease in general. For example, fat intake has increased from 10% of total energy intake for adult Japanese in the 1960s to 25% by the 2000s, and mean serum cholesterol levels have increased from approximately 150–160 mg/dL to 200–210 mg/dL during that same timeframe (Kitamura et al. 2008; Iso, 2008). Therefore, primary prevention for hypertension, diabetes, smoking, and dyslipidemia from early in the life course should be strengthened.

Conclusion

Japan has been successful in reducing stroke mortality over the past few decades, starting with a program originating in Ikawa town, Akita Prefecture in 1963. The most successful elements of this community-based program were the regular health checkups and targeted health promotion campaigns which promoted and normalized healthy lifestyles. The program was implemented via a network of multidisciplinary health professionals, including physicians, public health nurses, nutritionists, clerical workers, and researchers.

References

Central Intelligence Agency (CIA). (2016). *CIA World Factbook*. Retrieved March 14, 2018, from https://www.cia.gov/library/publications/the-world-factbook/.
Heifetz, RA., Linsky, M. (2002). Leadership on the Line. Boston: Harvard Business School Press.
Iso, H. (2008). Changes in coronary heart disease risk among Japanese. *Circulation, 118*, 2725–2729.
Iso, H., Shimamoto, T., Naito, Y., Sato, S., Kitamura, A., & Iida, M. (1998). Effects of a long-term hypertension control program on stroke incidence and prevalence in a rural community in Northeastern Japan. *Stroke, 29*(8), 1510–1518.
Komachi, K. (2007). *Epidemiological studies of cardiovascular disease and development of community-based prevention programs. 40-year histories in Akita and Osaka*. Tokyo: Japan Public Health Association Press. (in Japanese).

Kubo, M., et al. (2003). Trends in the incidence, mortality, and survival of cardiovascular disease in a Japanese community: the Hisayama study. *Stroke, 34*, 2349–2354.

Kitamura, A., Sato, S., Kiyama, M., Imano, H., Iso, H., Okada, T., Ohira, T., Tanigawa, T., Yamagishi, K., Nakamura, M., Konishi, M., Shimamoto, T., Iida, M., & Komachi, Y. (2008). Trends in the incidence of coronary heart disease and stroke and their risk factors in Japan, 1964 to 2003: the Akita-Osaka study. *Journal of the American College of Cardiology, 52*(1), 71–79. https://doi.org/10.1016/j.jacc.2008.02.075.

Liu, L., Ikeda, K., & Yamori, Y. (2001). Changes in stroke mortality rates for 1950 to 1997. A great slowdown of decline trend in Japan. *Stroke, 32*, 1745–1749.

Nomura, S., Sakamoto, H., Glenn, S., Tsugawa, Y., Abe, S. K., & Rahman, M. M. (2017). Population health and regional variations of disease burden in Japan, 1990-2015: a systematic subnational analysis for the Global Burden of disease study 2015. *Lancet, 390*, 1521–1538.

Ozawa, H. (1968). Death and incidence rates of cerebrovascular disease in Akita and Osaka. *Japanese Journal of Public Health, 15*, 23–32. (in Japanese).

Sarti, C., Rastenyte, D., Cepaitis, Z., & Tuomilehto, J. (2000). International trends in mortality from stroke, 1968 to 1994. *Stroke, 31*, 1588–1601.

Shimamoto, T., Iso, H., Sankai, T., Iida, M., Naito, Y., Sato, S., (1994). Can blood pressure in the elderly be reduced? Findings from a long-term population survey in Japan. *The American Journal of Geriatric Cardiology*, 42–50.

Shimamoto, T., Komachi, Y., Inada, H., Doi, M., Iso, H., & Sato, S. (1989). Trends for coronary heart disease and stroke and their risk factors in Japan. *Circulation, 79*(3), 503–515.

Ueshima, H. (2007). Explanation for the Japanese paradox: Prevention of increase in coronary heart disease and reduction in stroke. *Journal of Atherosclerosis and Thrombosis, 14*, 278–286.

United Nations Development Programme (UNDP). (2016). *Human Development Report 2016*. Retrieved March 14, 2018, from http://hdr.undp.org/sites/default/files/2016_human_development_report.pdf

Whelton, P. K., Carey, R. M., Aronow, W. S., Casey, D. E., Collins, K. J., & Himmelfarb, C. H. (2017). ACC/AHA/AAPA/ABC/ACPM/AGS/APhA/ASH/ASPC/NMA/PCNA Guideline for the prevention, detection, evaluation, and management of high blood pressure in adults - A report of the American College of Cardiology/American Heart Association Task Force on Clinical Practice Guidelines. *Journal of the American College of Cardiology, 71*(19), e127–e248. https://doi.org/10.1016/j.jacc.2017.11.006

World Health Organization (WHO). (2013). *Community-based efforts to reduce blood pressure and stroke in Japan*. Retrieved March 14, 2018, from http://www.who.int/features/2013/japan_blood_pressure/en/

World Health Organization (WHO). (2014). *Noncommunicable Diseases (NCD) Country Profiles: Japan*. Retrieved February 28, 2018, from http://www.who.int/nmh/countries/jpn_en.pdf?ua=1

World Health Organization (WHO). (2015). *Japan: WHO statistical profile*. Retrieved February 28, 2018, from http://www.who.int/gho/countries/jpn.pdf?ua=1

World Health Organization (WHO). (2017). *The top 10 causes of death*. Retrieved February 28, 2018, from http://www.who.int/mediacentre/factsheets/fs310/en/

Yamagishi, K., Sato, S., Kitamura, A., Kiyama, M., Okada, T., & Tanigawa, T. (2012). Cost-effectiveness and budget impact analyses of a long-term hypertension detection and control program for stroke prevention. *Journal of Hypertension, 30*(9), 1874–1879. https://doi.org/10.1097/HJH.0b013e3283568781

Yuzuki, K. (1958). Observation of adjusted mortality of vascular damage in central nervous system by prefecture. *Japanese Journal of Public Health, 5*, 299. (in Japanese).

Discussion Questions

1. What factors might help explain why Japan has such a serious problem with high blood pressure and stroke?
2. Why was it important to screen people as young as 30 years old for high blood pressure?
3. How are social determinants of health related to cerebrovascular disease (stroke)? How did this case address some of the most relevant social determinants in this community?
4. How was community ownership of this program promoted?
5. How have larger societal changes (such as modernization) over the past few decades helped or inhibited stroke prevention in Japan? What about in other countries?

Follow-Up Reading

World Health Organization. (2017). *The top 10 causes of death*. Retrieved from http://www.who.int/mediacentre/factsheets/fs310/en/.

World Health Organization. (2013). *Community-based efforts to reduce blood pressure and stroke in Japan*. Retrieved from http://www.who.int/features/2013/japan_blood_pressure/en/.

Yamagishi, K., Sato, S., Kitamura, A., Kiyama, M., Okada, T., Tanigawa, T., Iso, H. (2012). Cost-effectiveness and budget impact analyses of a long-term hypertension detection and control program for stroke prevention. *Journal of Hypertension*, *30*(9), 1874–79.

Chapter 6
Addressing Elder Abuse and Neglect in a Greying Malaysia: The PEACE Initiative

Raudah Mohd Yunus, Noran Naqiah Hairi, Choo Wan Yuen, Farizah Hairi, Sajaratulnisah Othman, Siti Zaharah Jamaluddin, Devi Peramalah, Zainudin Mohd Ali, and Awang Bulgiba

Malaysia: Demographics Overview
Population: 31,381,992
Life expectancy: 75 years

- Male: 72.2
- Female: 78

GNI per capita: $24,620
Total fertility rate: 2.5 children/woman
Under-five mortality rate: 9
UN HDI: 0.789
Top three causes of death

- Ischemic heart disease
- Stroke
- Lower respiratory infections

Source: WHO publications (2015)

R. M. Yunus (✉)
Department of Social and Preventive Medicine, University of Malaya, Kuala Lumpur, Malaysia

Department of Public Health, Faculty of Medicine, Sungai Buloh Campus, Universiti Teknologi Mara (UiTM), Sungai Buloh, Malaysia

N. N. Hairi · C. W. Yuen · F. Hairi · D. Peramalah · A. Bulgiba
Department of Social and Preventive Medicine, University of Malaya, Kuala Lumpur, Malaysia

S. Othman
Department of Primary Care Medicine, University Malaya Medical Centre, Kuala Lumpur, Malaysia

© Springer Nature Switzerland AG 2019
M. Withers, J. McCool (eds.), *Global Health Leadership*,
https://doi.org/10.1007/978-3-319-95633-6_6

History

Malaysia is undergoing a rapid demographic transition. The subject of abuse and exploitation of older adults gained national spotlight in the late 1990s. A number of newspaper headlines on abuse and abandonment of older adults (Harian, 2012; Utusan, 1998) had triggered public outcries, prompting national debates on the vulnerability of senior citizens. This concern was later reflected in the 8th Malaysian Plan (2001–2005) which emphasized older adults' welfare and protection. The issue was again manifested in the subsequent 9th (2006–2010) and 10th Malaysian Plan (2011–2015). These developments collectively created a window of opportunity to establish a platform where stakeholders could work together in combating elder abuse and neglect (EAN), and through which the **P**revent **E**lder **A**buse and negle**C**t initiativ**E** (PEACE) was born.

Given that a culture of respect, obedience, and care for parents and elderly family members is strongly ingrained within Malaysian society (Talib & Jamaluddin, 2014), EAN has traditionally been considered taboo. There is a tendency among family members and victims to hide their abuse experiences due to fear of stigma (Acierno, 2003). Similarly, community members tend to avoid intervening in what is regarded as a "private matter." On the other hand, ageism— the stereotyping and prejudice against older persons—has not been adequately explored and understood in the Malaysian context. Current existing literature on ageism, derived mainly from western countries (Liu, Norman, & While, 2013), is relevant to Malaysia as it transitions toward becoming an upper-middle income country with changing social norms and values (Aziz & Yusooff, 2012). For example, the notion that old age is affiliated with stereotypes such as "burdensome," "unproductive," "nearly dying," and "backward" was previously uncommon. In addition, there is a growing concern that Malaysian elders are being marginalized, with almost one-half reported to be at risk of social isolation (Ibrahim, Abolfathi Momtaz, & Hamid, 2013).

Nevertheless, the trend in elder abuse has gradually changed over the past several years; EAN has received increasing media coverage thus sparking greater interest among various stakeholders to look into the subject more seriously. A local study found that among rural elders, (the prevalence of EAN (from the age of 60) stood at 8.1%, with financial abuse and psychological abuse being the most common subtypes – 4.8% and 3.4% respectively) (Yunus et al., 2016). When strangers as perpetrators were included in the definition of abuse, financial abuse doubled, pushing the overall prevalence of EAN to 13.6% (Yunus et al., 2016).

S. Z. Jamaluddin
Faculty of Law, University of Malaya, Kuala Lumpur, Malaysia

Z. M. Ali
State Health Department of Negeri Sembilan, Seremban, Negeri Sembilan, Malaysia

Introduction

Demographics and Economy

Malaysia is an upper-middle income country with approximately 32 million people. The major ethnic Malay group consists of 68.8% of total population, whereas Chinese comprised 23.2%, Indians 7%, and others 1% (DoSM, 2017). Its gross domestic product (GDP)—a measure of national income and output—was estimated at US$296 billion in 2016, representing 0.48% of the world economy. The country today is one of the leading exporters of electrical appliances, electrical parts and components, and natural gas (World Bank, 2017).

Health in Malaysia

According to WHO, life expectancy in Malaysia as of 2015 was 73 for men and 77 for women. Health expenditure ranges between 4 and 5% of the country's GDP. The top five leading causes of death in Malaysia are ischemic heart disease, stroke, lower respiratory infections, road traffic injuries, and chronic obstructive pulmonary disease. From 1990 to 2013, the under-five mortality rate dropped from 17 to 9 per 1000 live births, while the maternal mortality ratio decreased from 56 to 29 per 100,000 live births (WHO, 2015). According to the Malaysian Department of Statistics in 2015, those aged 60 years or older comprised 9.13% of the population. However, this figure is expected to increase to 15% by 2030 (Manaf, Omar, Omar, & Salleh, 2017) and 17.6% by 2040 (United Nations, 2015).

Health Impacts of EAN

Various studies have documented the adverse health impacts of abuse in late life. EAN does not only affect physical health but also psychological, social, and behavioral health. A systematic review on the consequences of EAN ranked premature mortality as the most consistent and credible outcome, followed by depressive symptomatology and anxiety. EAN has been demonstrated to cause higher rates of healthcare utilization, disability, and numerous negative physical and mental health-related symptoms (Yunus et al., 2017).

Description of the Program

The Program: Prevent Elder Abuse and Neglect (PEACE)

In response to the growing dilemma of EAN in Malaysia, the Prevent Elder Abuse and negleCt initiativE (PEACE) was commenced in early 2014, in line with the vision of the National Health Policy for Older Persons (2008) and National Policy for Older Persons (2011). These two policies were introduced by the Malaysian government as a result of the rapid demographic transition, in order to address issues related to senior citizens. The overarching aims of these two policies were (1) formulation of strategies which safeguard older adults' rights and welfare; (2) promotion and advocacy of issues relevant to older adults; (3) encouragement of lifelong learning, active participation in community activities, and intergenerational solidarity; and (4) promotion of strong governance and shared responsibility among stakeholders. PEACE is a five-package program which aims at advancing EAN research and services through a coordinated, multistep approach involving stakeholders across sectors.

Program Objectives

Specific objectives of PEACE programs were as follows:

1. To examine the magnitude, risk factors, and consequences of EAN among community dwellers and institutionalized older adults
2. To investigate the role of caregiver strain in preventing EAN
3. To provide education and training to healthcare providers
4. To provide education and training to formal and informal caregivers
5. To identify existing laws on EAN, understand the gaps, and refine them via a more comprehensive approach

Program Stakeholders

A multi-sectoral partnership was formed in order to implement PEACE. This involved (1) academics and clinicians from different disciplines including public health, family medicine, geriatrics and law; (2) officials from the state health department; (3) the Department of Social Welfare; (4) various community-based organizations; and (5) media outlets. Negeri Sembilan, one of the fourteen states in Malaysia, was chosen for the pilot phase, and programs were then gradually expanded to other states.

Table 6.1 EAN programs and outcomes

Activity/project	Type	Objective/outcome
Community engagement	Training program for institutional caregivers (CG) in Seremban	Improvement of skills and knowledge among CG
	Training on EAN intervention for healthcare providers	Improvement of skills and knowledge among doctors and nurses
	National Senior Citizens Day and public forums	Increased public awareness
	World Elder Abuse Awareness Week	Increased public awareness
	Interviews with local news outlets	Increase of public awareness
Research	Observational studies 1. Elder mistreatment in a community-dwelling population: the Malaysian Elder Mistreatment Project (MAESTRO) (Choo et al., 2016) 2. Physical function and disability among elderly living in rural community 3. Need assessment for caregivers of elderly living in rural community 4. Systematic review on EAN interventions (Choo, Hairi, Othman, Francis, & Baker, 2013) 5. Understanding of EAN among healthcare professionals (Ahmed et al., 2016) Intervention studies 1. Educational intervention to reduce burden and stress among caregivers 2. Improving nurses' detection and management of EAN (I-NEED) (Loh et al., 2015) 3. An educational intervention on improving detection and management of EAN among doctors	

Program Outcomes

To date, a number of positive results have been obtained from the successful implementation of both academic and community engagement activities, while some programs are still in progress. Some of the major programs and accomplishments of PEACE are summarized in Table 6.1. PEACE activities include different types of community engagement, awareness-raising campaigns such as the National Senior Citizens Day and World Elder Abuse Awareness Week, and training of caregivers and healthcare providers. Other than that, research is a key component of PEACE, aiming at gathering baseline information about the subject and developing effective interventions.

Key Components of Leadership

The implementation of PEACE involved multiple partners and stakeholders at various levels. Challenges therefore were inevitable, making effective leadership central to the smooth and successful execution of programs, and accomplishment of the objectives. Some key components of leadership are discussed below.

Vision

PEACE started with a clear vision of reducing the burden of EAN in Malaysia. A well-defined and realistic vision is the first and most important criteria in any endeavor. In this case, by first laying out the vision in a visually presentable manner and communicating it to potential partners, people were mobilized from across disciplines and sectors. Clarity of vision was crucial as a guide to undertake the next steps: formulation of strategies, implementation of programs, monitoring, and evaluation. Whenever complacency or conflicts emerged, a clear and shared vision was often the stronger force that united all stakeholders.

Team Building

Given the cross-sectoral and cross-disciplinary nature of PEACE stakeholders, building a mutual understanding and cooperation among all partners was extremely important. Regular team building programs in the form of communication, decision-making, planning activities and games were carried out. Team building strengthened the relationships between different groups, made implementation smoother by avoiding conflicts, fostered trust and the spirit of collectivism, gave a sense of reward and satisfaction to individuals, and promoted exchange of ideas and knowledge transfer. In addition, team building facilitated efforts to capitalize on the diversity of talents and enhanced understanding of each other's characteristics and working styles.

Communication Skills

While undertaking the various initiatives of PEACE, effective communications skills were critical in every step, particularly in the following: (a) while engaging with different stakeholders who may not share similar perspectives; (b) while reaching out to the public to convey the message of the programs; (c) while translating the work and findings onto papers—be it popular writings or academic articles; and (d) while giving recommendations to the higher authority with regard to policies and legislations. On the contrary, poor communication posed the risks of creating unnecessary misunderstandings, forming barriers to the acceptance of good ideas, and causing easily preventable rejection or backlash from the higher authority or other stakeholders. The following steps were employed to ensure good communication: (1) formulating a communication strategy, (2) developing a communication process, and (3) facilitating and encouraging feedback.

Innovation and Flexibility

As the PEACE initiative was the first of its kind in Malaysia, it was difficult to predict or anticipate upcoming hurdles. Various obstacles—such as financial constraint, shortage of human resource, impediments in data collection, and other logistical issues—taught the team to perform trial and error, experiment with new things, and continuously innovate the programs, techniques, and approaches. The need for flexibility and innovation is indisputable, and it is important that health leaders have this understanding in mind before embarking on any project. As much as a carefully planned schedule and timeline has been set, room for change and adaptability must exist.

Managing the Human Factor

Addressing the human factor—defined as human physical and psychological behavior—was the most challenging part in this project. This was due to the diverse nature of our stakeholders and workforce which naturally created differences in personality, opinion, working style, expectations, priorities, interests, and needs. Values like respect, empathy, tolerance, and understanding were extremely vital in order to avoid unnecessary disputes or tension which could hamper the work. Effective management of individuals is a core ingredient in producing future health leaders who are motivated and competent.

Future Directions

PEACE is envisioned as an impetus for a more extensive multilevel, nationwide effort for the protection of elders in Malaysia. Ongoing effort and future plans are being made to expand this project, which include the following.

Focusing on Financial Abuse as One of the EAN Subtypes Needing Urgent Intervention

Our findings have demonstrated that financial exploitation the most common subtype of EAN. Similarly, financial abuse had the highest correlation with mortality among Malaysian elders, indicating its severity of impact on health and well-being. One possible explanation is that financial deprivation limits older adults' mobility, access to healthcare, and purchasing power—which can all contribute to social isolation, deterioration of living condition, and worsening of existing illnesses (Yunus et al., 2017). The growing virtual transactions such as internet and mobile banking (with continuous evolution) and little awareness among financial institutions are expected to intensify this problem. Future interventions will take a more holistic approach by (a) providing financial management skills and services for older adults, (b) formulating strategies to reduce the likelihood of financial manipulation through virtual transactions involving senior citizens, and (c) advocating for laws to prevent scams and similar activities from targeting older adults.

Prioritizing Institutionalized Older Adults in Future Programs

Older adults in institutional care have been relatively neglected in research despite existing evidence of their vulnerability to abuse. There is a need in the future to engage home care residents in community programs and research projects.

Improvement and Transformation of Healthcare Services

Healthcare providers involved in the PEACE initiative play the roles of conducting research and training other health personnel. A pilot training session has been conducted in one state among a group of selected physicians. This educational intervention will be replicated in other states to involve a larger number of doctors and nurses if it is effective. The goal is to incorporate EAN into daily clinical practice at primary health care facilities, develop standard clinical guidelines in EAN management and establish a reporting system. Hopefully, this will gradually push for bigger transformations in health services to accommodate for future health system demands.

Legal Strategy and Human Rights Approach

The two existing national policies on older adults are rather comprehensive. However, the gap lies in enforcement and implementation. From the legal perspective, older Malaysians are not fully protected from abuse. The PEACE project thus aims at pushing for more effective legislations either by amending the existing, relevant acts, or passing a new act which is specific to elder abuse. To achieve this, engagement with legal experts, legislators, and policy-makers is necessary. In addition, addressing EAN from the human rights perspective is not yet a common practice in Malaysia. Plans to strengthen elder protection using the right to health approach are needed (Friedman & Gostin, 2012; Yamin, 2005).

Combating Ageism

Most activities under the PEACE initiative to date have not directly addressed ageism. In the next phase, we will attempt to address this subject through different approaches such as positive media portrayal of elders and incorporation of elder-related issues into the school syllabus (Langer, 1999; North & Fiske, 2012).

Conclusion

The PEACE initiative describes how effective leaderhip skills are essential in any health agenda. These skills include identifying the right problem, building a clear vision for action, engaging key stakeholders, developing teamwork, decision-making and problem-solving. Conflicts, whether interpersonal or interorganizational, are bound to arise and could disrupt actual tasks and goals. Without effective leadership, a vision remains a vision. The five key leadership components discussed in this chapter— vision, team building, communication skills, innovation and flexibility, and managing the human factors—were highly relevant to PEACES experiences and will be useful as a guide for those who are planning to embark on future health-related projects.

References

Acierno, R. (2003). *Elder mistreatment: Epidemiological assessment methodology. Abuse, neglect and exploitation in an aging America.* Washington DC: National Academies Press.

Ahmed, A., Choo, W. Y., Othman, S., Hairi, N. N., Hairi, F. M., & Mohd Mydin, F. H. (2016). Understanding of elder abuse and neglect among health care professionals in Malaysia: An exploratory survey. *Journal of Elder Abuse & Neglect, 28*(3), 163–177.

Aziz, R. A., & Yusooff, F. (2012). Intergenerational relationships and communication among the rural aged in Malaysia. *Asian Social Science, 8*(6), 184.

Choo, W.Y., Hairi, N.N., Othman, S., Francis, D.P., Baker, P.R. (2013). *Interventions for preventing abuse in the elderly.* The Cochrane Library. Retrieved March 7, 2018, from http://onlinelibrary. wiley.com/doi/10.1002/14651858.CD010321.pub2/full

Choo, W. Y., Hairi, N. N., Sooryanarayana, R., Yunus, R. M., Hairi, F. M., & Ismail, N. (2016). Elder mistreatment in a community dwelling population: the Malaysian Elder Mistreatment Project (MAESTRO) cohort study protocol. *BMJ Open, 6*(5), e011057.

Department of Statistics Malaysia. (2017). Population & demography. Retrieved March 7, 2018, from https://www.dosm.gov.my.

Friedman, E. A., & Gostin, L. O. (2012). Pillars for progress on the right to health: Harnessing the potential of human rights through a framework convention on Global Health. *Health and Human Rights, 14*(1), 4–19.

Harian, B. (2012) *Nasib Ayah Nyanyuk.* Semasa. Retrieved March 7, 2018, from http://eresources. nlb.gov.sg/newspapers/digitised/issue/beritaharian20010111-1.

Ibrahim, R., Abolfathi Momtaz, Y., & Hamid, T. A. (2013). Social isolation in older Malaysians: Prevalence and risk factors. *Psychogeriatrics, 13*(2), 71–79.

Langer, N. (1999). Changing youngsters' perception of aging: Aging education's role. *Educational Gerontology, 25*(6), 549–554.

Liu, Y. E., Norman, I. J., & While, A. E. (2013). Nurses' attitudes towards older people: A systematic review. *International Journal of Nursing Studies, 50*(9), 1271–1282.

Loh, D. A., Choo, W. Y., Hairi, N. N., Othman, S., Mohd Hairi, F., & Mydin, M. (2015). A cluster randomized trial on improving nurses' detection and management of elder abuse and neglect (I-NEED): Study protocol. *Journal of Advanced Nursing, 71*(11), 2661–2672.

Manaf, N. H. A., Omar, A., Omar, M. A., & Salleh, M. (2017). Determinants of healthcare utilisation among the elderly in Malaysia. *Institutions and Economies, 9*, 115–140.

North, M. S., & Fiske, S. T. (2012). An inconvenienced youth? Ageism and its potential intergenerational roots. *Psychological Bulletin, 138*(5), 982.

Talib, N, Jamaluddin, S. (2014). *The search for well-being through policies, system and values.* Retrieved March 8, 2018, from https://doi.org/10.2139/ssrn.2466793

Utusan. (1998). *Warga Tua Kenapa Mereka Diabaikan? Gaya Hidup.* Retrieved December 19, 2017, from http://ww1.utusan.com.my/utusan/info.asp?y=1998&dt=0106&pub=Utusan_Malaysia&sec=Gaya_Hidup&pg=ls_01.htm

United Nations, Department of Economic and Social Affairs, Population Division (2015). World population prospects: The 2015 Revision. Retrieved from http://esa.un.org/unpd/wpp/DVD

World Bank (2017). *The World Bank in Malaysia: Overview.* Retrieved December 19, 2017, from www.worldbank.org/en/country/malaysia/overview

World Health Organization (WHO) (2015). *Countries.* Retrieved December 19, 2017, from http://www.who.int/countries/mys/en/.

Yamin, A. E. (2005). The right to health under international law and its relevance to the United States. *American Journal of Public Health, 95*(7), 1156–1161.

Yunus, R. M., Hairi, N. N., Choo, W. Y., Hairi, F. M., Sooryanarayana, R., & Ahmad, S. N. (2016). Mortality among elder abuse victims in rural Malaysia: A two-year population-based descriptive study. *Journal of Elder Abuse & Neglect, 29*(1), 59–71.

Yunus, R. M., Hairi, N. N., Choo, W. Y., Hairi, F. M., Sooryanarayana, R., & Ahmad, S. N. (2017). Mortality among elder abuse victims in rural Malaysia: A two-year population-based descriptive study. *Journal of Elder Abuse & Neglect, 29*(1), 59–71.

Discussion Questions

1. Describe in brief the demographic transition that is happening in developing countries and how it might escalate the phenomenon of elder abuse and neglect (EAN).
2. In your opinion, why did elder abuse receive relatively little (or late) attention as compared to other forms of family violence such as intimate partner violence (IPV) and child abuse?
3. How does ageism contribute to EAN? Does the pathway differ between developed and developing countries?
4. What are the advantages and disadvantages of addressing EAN from the human rights perspective compared to other conventional approaches?
5. List five additional leadership components that you feel are relevant to this case (other than the five mentioned). How would you apply these components in another health-related project?

Follow-Up Reading

Williams, J. L., Hernandez-Tejada, M. A., & Acierno, R. (2016). *24 elder abuse: Prevention and reporting.* The Oxford Handbook of Behavioral Emergencies and Crises, 373.

Pillemer, K., Burnes, D., Riffin, C., & Lachs, M. S. (2016). Elder abuse: Global situation, risk factors, and prevention strategies. *The Gerontologist, 56*(Suppl 2), S194-S205.

Du Mont, J., Macdonald, S., Kosa, D., Elliot, S., Spencer, C., & Yaffe, M. (2015). Development of a Comprehensive Hospital-Based Elder Abuse Intervention: An Initial Systematic Scoping Review. *PloS One, 10*(5), e0125105.

Dong, X. (2016). Elder Abuse in Nursing Homes: How Do We Advance the Field of Elder Justice?. *Annals of Internal Medicine, 165*(4), 288-289.

North, M. S., & Fiske, S. T. (2012). An inconvenienced youth? Ageism and its potential intergenerational roots. *Psychological Bulletin, 138*(5), 982.

Chapter 7
Community Engagement in Maternal and Newborn Health in Eastern Indonesia

Salut Muhidin, Rachmalina Prasodjo, Maria Silalahi, and Jerico F. Pardosi

Indonesia: Demographics Overview
Population: 260,580,739
Life expectancy: 72.7 years

- Male: 70.1
- Female: 75.5

GNI per capita: $10,053
Total fertility rate: 2.11 children/woman
Under-five mortality rate (per 1000 live births): 29
UN HDI: 0.689
Top three causes of death

- Stroke
- Ischaemic heart disease
- Diabetes mellitus

Source: CIA World Factbook (2016), UNDP Human Development Programme (2016), WHO publications (2015)

S. Muhidin (✉)
Macquarie University in Sydney, Sydney, NSW, Australia
e-mail: salut.muhidin@mq.edu.au

R. Prasodjo
National Institute of Health Research and Development (NIHRD),
The Ministry of Health-Indonesia, Central Jakarta, Indonesia

M. Silalahi
Community Health Division, Nusa Tengarra Timur (NTT) Provincial Health,
Kota Kupang, Nusa Tenggara Timur, Indonesia

J. F. Pardosi
School of Public Health and Community Medicine, University of New South Wales (UNSW),
Sydney, NSW, Australia

© Springer Nature Switzerland AG 2019
M. Withers, J. McCool (eds.), *Global Health Leadership*,
https://doi.org/10.1007/978-3-319-95633-6_7

Studies have indicated that a combination of clinical- and community-based interventions has the potential to reduce maternal and infant mortality in low- and middle-income countries (Farnsworth et al., 2014; Hamer et al., 2015; Piane, 2009). Community-based health interventions, by definition, often involve active partnerships with multiple stakeholders within and across a community. The main reason for using a community engagement approach is based on the assumption that behaviour (including health and illness) is shaped by social and physical environments. If health is understood to be socially determined, health issues are therefore best addressed by engaging all community members who can bring their understanding of the community and its unique health challenged to a project. Community engagement typically encompasses a variety of activities from information sharing to community empowerment and collaborative or shared leadership. Shared leadership is vital in that it can facilitate the community engagement process in a number of ways, including achieving the main goal of engagement (which is to build trusting, mutually beneficial relationships), enlisting and utilizing new resources and allies, creating effective communication channels and improving overall health outcomes as projects evolve into lasting collaborations (Shore, 2007).

Building on the conceptual and theoretical aspects of leadership developed in previous research, this chapter examines the importance of leadership in improving maternal and newborn health. More specifically, it investigates the concept of shared leadership among stakeholders in community engagement programs to improve maternal and newborn health in the Eastern province of Indonesia, Nusa Tenggara Timur. The case study illustrates how a shared leadership model increased the level of community engagement, a key facet in the success of the program. The lessons learned can be used in various contexts in which the programs may involve a culture of collaboration within the community.

Introduction

High rates of maternal and child mortality remain persistent in many low- and middle-income countries (LMICs), including Indonesia. The United Nations, through its Sustainable Development Goals (SDGs), provides high level guidance to all countries, in particular LMICs to achieve substantial reductions in their maternal and child mortality rates. Specifically, the third SDG states the goal of reducing the global maternal mortality ratio to less than 70 per 100,000 live births by 2030. At the same time, all countries are advised to end preventable deaths of newborns and children under 5 years of age by reducing neonatal mortality rate to a minimum of 12 per 1000 live births and the under-five mortality rate to a minimum of 25 per 1000 live births (UN, 2017). Accordingly, Indonesia has made a strong commitment to address this issue especially among its eastern regions where these mortality rates are among the highest in the country. The Nusa Tenggara Timur (NTT) province has a maternal mortality ratio (MMR) of 307 per 100,000 live births and an infant mortality rate (IMR) of 45 per 1000 live births, which compares poorly to the national Indonesian statistics of 239 per 100,000 and 32 per 1000, respectively (Statistics Indonesia et al., 2013). However, this province is not unique in its need to address high rates of maternal and infant deaths; it represents the situation of many rural communities in Eastern Indonesia (Pardosi, Parr, & Muhidin, 2017). The majority of childbirths in that region take place at home (57.4%), and complications during pregnancy and childbirth are one of the major causes of maternal and newborn mortality.

Pregnant women face considerate risk giving birth at home. This decision is often mediated by prior experience and the reality of their immediate environment (Rajendra, Svend, and Birgitte (2004)), for example, indicated that low socio-economic status is a factor influencing the preference for home births in India. Other factors that may increase the likelihood of giving birth at home include beginning labour at night, beliefs that home birth is safer, health workers negative attitudes or discrimination and fears of medical interventions (Boucher, Bennett, McFarlin, & Freeze, 2009; Mwifadhi et al., 2007; Ravi & Ravishankar, 2014). Studies also report geographical distance, and poor road conditions are other reasons why mothers may prefer home deliveries (Thaddeus & Maine, 1994; Titaley, Hunter, Dibley, & Heywood, 2010). In their meta-analysis, Finlayson and Downe (2013) concluded that a misalignment between antenatal care provision and the sociocultural context is the main driver for underutilization of health services in low- and middle-income countries.

Thaddeus and Maine (1994) in their early work proposed that maternal mortality is related to three delays (Fig. 7.1.). The first delay is recognizing the problem and deciding to seek care. Factors shaping this decision-making process include knowledge about pregnancy and childbirth complications, recognizing the seriousness of symptoms, cultural beliefs, and traditional decision-making roles. The second delay is reaching a health facility, which is often related to physical accessibility factors such as geographical distance from the health facility and the availability and cost of transportation. The third delay is receiving adequate and appropriate care. Availability of supplies and equipment, a lack of trained and

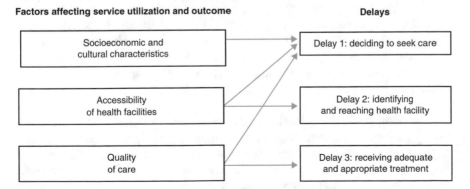

Fig. 7.1 The Three Delays Model. Source: Thaddeus & Maine, 1994

competent personnel, and the quality of care received all contribute to this delay. Even today, the "Three Delays Model" is used to explain what causes maternal deaths in many developing country settings, including in the Indonesian context.

Levels of Intervention

The literature indicates that there are variations in defining the concepts of collaborative or shared leadership. It generally focuses on the need to broadly distribute the tasks and responsibilities of leadership up, down and across the hierarchy of stakeholders. Shared leadership offers a concept of leadership practice as a group- or team-level phenomenon in which leaders aim to communicate to achieve collaboration and the achievement of team goals (Liang & Sandmann, 2015; Pearce & Conger, 2002). Thus, shared leadership can be differentiated from what is traditionally found in a hierarchical organization in that participation is voluntary and egalitarian. Shared leadership often entails cooperation by involved organizations with different cultures and agendas. In the context of health programs, Alexander, Comfort, Weiner and Bogue (2001) emphasized the importance of leadership in collaborative community health partnerships which can involve different stakeholders who are concerned with health-related issues. At the same time, many health programs are complex and multidimensional; shared leadership is significant and relevant in supporting heath programs.

Nevertheless, there are some challenges in implementing shared leadership. Alexander et al. (2001) pointed out three challenges: (1) the issues of continuity or change in partnership leadership, (2) the differences in leadership development stages, and (3) the issues of power and participation in a neutral shared leadership. First, a shared partnership may be disrupted or discontinued when there are any big changes in leadership. In order to achieve the long-term goals as agreed by involved stakeholders, continuity in leadership brings necessary stability. Second, shared leadership may involve different individuals who may also have different stages in their leadership roles and understanding. Some may already be in their later stages of leadership development, while others are still at the earlier stages in which mentoring and support are very much needed to facilitate their leadership roles. Third, shared leadership is built by assuming a neutral leadership among involved parties. It should foster equal voice and representation among all partners, regardless of differences in resources, power and size. This could be disrupted when one of the involved actors start to dominate or favour a particular constituency over the best interests of the collective.

Farnsworth et al. (2014) considered the importance of shared leadership, which usually happens in the latest stage of the community engagement process. Earlier stages of engagement are characterized as outreach, consult, involve and collaborate (Fig. 7.2). Community engagement is seen as a continuum of community collaborations that ideally lead to active engagement. Over time, a specific collaboration is likely to move along this continuum toward greater community

		Increasing Level of Community Involvement, Impact, Trust and Communication Flow ➤		
Outreach	**Consult**	**Involve**	**Collaborate**	**Shared Leadership**
Some Community Involvement	*More Community Involvement*	*Better Community Involvement*	*Community Involvement*	*Strong Bidirectional Relationship*
Communication flows from one to the other, to inform	*Communication flows to the community and then back, answer seeking*	*Communication flows both ways, participatory form of communication*	*Communication flow bidirectional*	*Final decision-making at community level*
Provides community with information	*Gets information or feedback from the community*	*Involves more participation with community on issues*	*Forms partnerships with community on each aspect of project from development to solution*	*Entities have formed strong partnership structures*
Entities coexist	*Entities share information*	*Entities cooperate with each other*	*Entities form bidirectional communication channels*	*Outcomes: Broader health outcomes affecting broader community; strong bidirectional trust built*
Outcomes: Optimally establishes communication channels and channels for outreach	*Outcomes: Develops connections*	*Outcomes: Visibility of partnership established with increased cooperation*	*Outcomes: Partnership building, trust building*	

Fig. 7.2 Types and levels of community engagement. Source: Farnsworth et al. (2014)

involvement. It also frequently evolves to long-term partnerships that move from the traditional focus on a single health issue to address a range of social, economic, political and environmental factors that affect community health.

Program Description

Current and Past Interventions in Indonesia

In 2009, the government of NTT implemented a progressive health program focused on maternal and child health called the "Revolusi Kesehatan Ibu dan Anak" (known as "Revolusi KIA"), which means "Mother and Child Health Revolution" (NTT Provincial Health Office, 2012). The program has two main objectives: (1) to save mothers and their babies during delivery through health facility births and (2) to improve the quality of health-care services through improvement and strengthening of health facilities. Without adequate medical equipment, even well-trained health workers cannot provide adequate medical care if they face an emergency situation, such as postpartum haemorrhage. For that reason, all mothers therefore are required to give birth in health facilities such as a community health centre (called a *puskesmas* in Indonesia) at the sub-district level or a hospital at the district and provincial levels. The *Revolusi KIA* health program was expected to help make significant reductions to maternal and child mortality rates by mandating population-level behavioural changes involving all stakeholders in the community, including individual caregivers, health staff, the government as well as general community members. In other words, collaboration among the stakeholders that involves sharing responsibilities was seen as a requirement to improve maternal and child health.

Outcomes of Community-Based Interventions

A number of studies on maternal and child health programs in Asia indicate that community engagement can improve maternal and child health by mobilizing people to use health facilities for childbirth and by building partnership with local leaders (Haines et al., 2007; Kerber et al., 2007; Rosato et al., 2008). In Cambodia, for example, community-based programs were supported by local community leaders, which led to higher child survival (Oum, Chandramohan, & Cairncross, 2005). A study in Indonesian West Java Province found that the local community leaders could successfully promote health programs, particularly to help women who experienced complications during childbirth (Titaley et al., 2010).

One of the most important components of the *Revolusi KIA* program is the referral health system called "the 2H2 Referral System". The 2H2 system aims to bring mothers from their homes to health facilities to have births and to return them back home safely. It is specifically defined as an intensive health monitoring program of pregnant women within 2 days before and 2 days after the due date (translated from the Bahasa Indonesian language: "2 Hari sebelum dan 2 Hari sesudah" or 2H2). The period of 2 days before and after delivery is considered a critical period, as most maternal deaths (90% in NTT province as of 2012) occur soon after delivery (IDHS in Statistics Indonesia et al., 2013). Thus, the 2H2 system aims to alert and mobilize all interested parties involved in the delivery to ensure that mothers give birth at an appropriate health facility. Although the referral system primarily focuses on the period of 2 days before and after delivery, monitoring actually begins at the first antenatal care visit by a village midwife.

Figure 7.3 indicates how community stakeholders at three different levels are involved in the 2H2 program. The first level consists of a pregnant woman and her family; the second level is the community, consisting of the neighbours, village

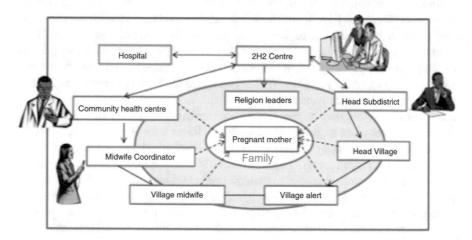

Fig. 7.3 Community work mechanism in the 2H2 system. Source: NTT Provincial Health Office (2012)

health volunteers, village midwife, traditional birth attendants and local community leaders; and the third level is government leaders and health facilitators, such as the 2H2 coordinator and hospital. In short, it is a combination of a clinical- and community-based intervention. The involvement of these parties begins when a pregnant woman is registered by the 2H2 Centre at the district level. The 2H2 Centre collects and monitors information relating to the health of pregnant women in the region, including the birth due dates, which is then shared with all relevant stakeholders in the community. This system aims to enhance efficiency through mobilizing those within the community who are willing and skilled to care for pregnant women and newborns.

Several strategies were used to drive the involvement of a variety of stakeholders in the 2H2 system, including verbal communication through multiple channels, a SMS or texts from mobile phones and the installation of a color-coded flag alert system in front of a pregnant woman's house. The flags are replaced regularly with different colours to signify different gestational stages of the unborn child. For example, a green flag is used for gestational age 0–3 months, a yellow flag for 4–6 months and a red flag for 7–9 months. By looking at the colour of the flag, it is expected anyone in the community would be able to help the pregnant woman and her family if there are any health problems during pregnancy, including taking her to the nearest health facility. In addition, a toll-free telephone number is available in case of emergency situations, such as unforeseen complications. Community stakeholders are asked to be prepared to support pregnant women in their region to have facility-based births.

Program Data Collection and Outcomes

To evaluate the impact of the program, a mixed-method data collection process was used. First, qualitative data were collected in 2014 in 12 health community centres at the sub-district level covering 6 representative districts in 3 main islands of NTT province: Flores, Sumba and West Timor. These were selected with equally inclusive criteria of easy and difficult or remote access to health centres. The data were collected by involving a combination of qualitative methods: in-depth interviews, focus group discussions (FGD) and roundtable discussions with health staff (from the district health office, local hospital, community health centre and village midwife), community leaders (i.e. the head of sub-district, the head of village and religious/community leader), other community members (i.e. traditional birth attendants/TBA) and family (mothers and family member). The purpose was to identify barriers and enabling factors in the implementation of the program. In total, 312 participants were asked about their knowledge, perceptions and attitudes regarding the health program and birthing practices (including home versus facility delivery). Once data were collected, they were transcribed and analysed through content and thematic analyses.

Table 7.1 Influencing factors in the implementation of 2H2 system in NTT, Indonesia

Reported barriers	Flores Timur	Sikka	Sumba Timur	SBD	TTS[a]	Belu
Knowledge of 2H2 system						
• Health providers	Moderate	Little	Moderate	Moderate	Little	Moderate
• Wider community	Moderate	Little	Little	Little	Little	Little
Financial						
• Economic reasons (poverty)	Moderate	Moderate	Strong/high	Moderate	Moderate	Moderate
Culture						
• Traditional practices	Moderate	Strong	Strong	Strong	Strong	Strong
• Roles of TBA	Little	Moderate	Strong	Little	Strong	Moderate
Health facilities and access						
• Not easy access	Moderate	Moderate	Moderate	Moderate	Moderate	Moderate
• Not enough facilities	Little	Moderate	Moderate	Moderate	Moderate	Little

[a]The program had just begun in TTS

Four common barriers in the implementation of 2H2 system were identified. These are knowledge of 2H2 system, financial issues, culture and health access (Table 7.1.). The level of influence of each barrier was also measured: "little" meant that less than 30% of participants felt that it was a barrier, "moderate" meant that 31–70% of participants felt it was a barrier, and "strong" signified more than 70% of participants felt it was a barrier to the implementation of the 2H2 system.

The 2H2 system had many challenges in terms of implementation, both from health providers and the community. For example, while most of the community members know about the importance of health facility births, some of them claimed that they never heard about this system. Among those who were involved, not all involved parties in all regions fully understood the essential elements of the program. They had not received adequate information on training on the steps of the program. Others perceived the program as health-related and did not engage with the program. While most acknowledged that they had an important role in helping mothers at the time of birth, most still believed that the major responsibility for assisting mothers was held by traditional birth attendants (TBA), especially among those who lived farthest away from health facilities. In some regions, the program was simply an intensive monitoring to a mother within 2 days before and 2 days after the delivery date, but it did not involve all stakeholders in the community.

Table 7.2 summarizes the responses from participants about their perceptions of the level of community engagement in each study area. The levels of barriers varied by study area and helped explain differences in levels of engagement. The communities within the districts were split into two categories according to ease of access to health facility, defined as the time and level of difficulty in reaching the closest health centre (travel time.) Communities that were located at least 1 h away by car from the nearest health centre were considered to be non-easy access. Despite differences in the levels of engagements in all districts, engagements in easy-access areas were perceived to be better than those in the non-easy access in all cases. This

Table 7.2 Level of community engagement for the 2H2 system in NTT-Indonesia

Districts and level of access to health facility	Outreach	Consult	Involve	Collaborate	Shared leadership
Flores Timur					
• Easy access region	0%	0%	27%	61%	12%
• Non-easy access region	29%	36%	29%	7%	0%
Sikka					
• Easy access region	43%	57%	0%	0%	0%
• Non-easy access region	40%	60%	0%	0%	0%
Sumba Timur					
• Easy access region	77%	23%	0%	0%	0%
• Non-easy access region	83%	17%	0%	0%	0%
Sumba Barat Daya					
• Easy access region	0%	41%	48%	11%	0%
• Non-easy access region	21%	59%	21%	0%	0%
Timor Tengah Selatan					
• Easy access region	74%	26%	0%	0%	0%
• Non-easy access region	100%	0%	0%	0%	0%
Belu					
• Easy access region	10%	21%	69%	0%	0%
• Non-easy access region	38%	62%	0%	0%	0%

implies that the accessibility can have an important impact on levels of engagement among community members.

Data from annual health reports collected by the NTT Health Office in 2014–2015 highlighted the success of the program. Since its implementation in 2010, improvements in health indicators have been observed. For example, in 2010 about 60% of pregnant women had facility births, and the provincial maternal mortality ratio (MMR) was 287 per 100,000. In 2011, 78% of pregnant women gave birth at a health facility, and the MMR decreased to 216 deaths per 100,000 live births (NTT PHO, 2012). At the district level, however, the rate of health facility births varied widely – from as low as 38% in South West Sumba to as high as 90% in Sikka during 2011. Those figures indicated that a large proportion of women in certain areas still did not give birth at the health facilities.

In the context of developing countries, economic reasons, cultural and traditional practices as well as the availability and access to health care have been cited as primary factors for why women do not give birth at health facilities. Even if a region has high levels of community engagement, the success of health facility birth program will be determined by other barriers. It is crucial to consider these barriers in each context and determine potential ways of responding. Some regions in Indonesia have had to modify the program based on their local challenges and requirements. For example, in communities where women are required to travel long distances or experience other difficulties in reaching health facilities, the program has been modified to start 5 or 7 days before and after the delivery due date.

Conclusion

Using the concept of community engagement as proposed by Farnsworth et al. (2014), this study reveals that community engagement in the NTT was mostly influenced by the level of shared leadership. Higher levels of community engagement occurred when close collaboration and shared leadership were present within the community. Accordingly, maternal and child health was significantly improved by actively mobilizing mothers and their families to use health facilities for births and through building partnership with the local governments. Leadership can be used as a primary enabling factor in transforming actions toward attaining health program's goals. Once a goal has been set, leaders must champion it in order to ensure that it will be achieved. In this case, leaders from all levels of community worked together toward a same broad, long-term vision for better health.

References

Alexander, J. A., Comfort, M. E., Weiner, B. J., & Bogue, R. (2001). Leadership in collaborative community health partnerships. *Nonprofit Management and Leadership, 12*, 159–175. https://doi.org/10.1002/nml.12203

Boucher, D., Bennett, C., McFarlin, B., & Freeze, R. (2009). Staying home to give birth; why women in the United States choose home birth. *Journal of Midwifery and Women's Health, 54*(2), 425–428.

CIA. (2016). *CIA World Factbook*. Retrieved March 14, 2018, from https://www.cia.gov/library/publications/the-world-factbook/

Farnsworth S.K, Böse K, Fajobi O, Souza P.P, Peniston A, Davidson L.L, et al. (2014). Community engagement to enhance child survival and early development in low- and middle-income countries: An evidence review. Journal of Health Communication, 19(sup 1), 67–88. doi: https://doi.org/10.1080/10810730.2014.941519.

Finlayson, K., & Downe, S. (2013). Why do women not use antenatal services in low- and middle-income countries? A meta-synthesis of qualitative studies. *PLoS Medicine, 10*(1), e1001373. https://doi.org/10.1371/journal.pmed.1001373

Haines, A., Sanders, D., Lehmann, U., Rowe, A. K., Lawn, J. E., & Jan, S. (2007). Achieving child survival goals: Potential contribution of community health workers. *Lancet, 369*(9579), 2121–2131.

Hamer, D. H., Herlihy, J. M., Musokotwane, K., Banda, B., Mpamba, C., Mwangelwa, B., et al. (2015). Engagement of the community, traditional leaders, and public health system in the design and implementation of a large community-based, cluster-randomized trial of umbilical cord care in Zambia. *American Journal of Tropical Medicine Hygiene, 92*(3), 666–672. https://doi.org/10.4269/ajtmh.14-0218

Kerber, K. J., de Graft-Johnson, J. E., Bhutta, Z. A., Okong, P., Starrs, A., & Lawn, J. E. (2007). Continuum of care for maternal, newborn, and child health: From slogan to service delivery. *Lancet, 370*, 1358–1369.

Liang, J. G., & Sandmann, L. R. (2015). Leadership for community engagement: A distributed leadership perspective. *Journal of Higher Education Outreach and Engagement, 19*(1), 35–63.

Mwifadhi, M., Joanna, A. S., Adiel, K. M., Brigit, O., Hassan, M., & Marcel, T. (2007). Factors affecting home delivery in rural Tanzani. *Tropical Medicine & International Health*. https://doi.org/10.1111/j.1365-3156.2007.01855

NTT Provincial Health Office. (2012). *Pedoman Revolusi KIA di Provinsi NTT [guidance of MCH revolution in Nusa Tenggara Timur Province], revised edition.* Kupang: NTT-PHO.

Oum, S., Chandramohan, C., & Cairncross, S. (2005). Community-based surveillance: A pilot study from rural Cambodia. *Tropical Medicine & International Health, 10*(7), 689–697.

Pardosi, J. F., Parr, N., & Muhidin, S. (2017). Local government and community leaders' perspectives on child health and mortality and inequity issues in rural eastern Indonesia. *Journal of Biosocial Science, 49*(1), 123–146. https://doi.org/10.1017/S0021932016000134

Pearce, C., & Conger, J. A. (Eds.). (2002). *Shared leadership: Reframing the how's and why's of leading others.* Thousand Oaks, CA: Sage Publishers.

Piane, G. M. (2009). Evidence-based practices to reduce maternal mortality: A systematic review. *Journal of Public Health, 31*(1), 26–31. https://doi.org/10.1093/pubmed/fdn074

Rajendra, R. W., Svend, S., & Birgitte, B. N. (2004). Socioeconomic and physical distance to the maternity hospital as predictors for place of delivery: An observation study from Nepal. *BMC Pregnancy and Childbirth, 4*, 8. https://doi.org/10.1186/1471-2393-4-8

Ravi, R. P., & Ravishankar, A. K. (2014). Does socio-demographic factors influence women's choice of place of delivery in rural areas of Tamilnadu state in India. *American Journal of Public Health Research, 2*(3), 75–80.

Rosato, M., Laverack, G., Grabman, L. H., Tripathy, P., Nair, N., & Mwansambo, C. (2008). Community participation: Lessons for maternal, newborn, and child health. *Lancet, 372*, 962–971.

Shore, N. (2007). Community-based participatory research and the ethics review process. *Journal of Empirical Research on Human Research Ethics, 2*(1), 31–41.

Statistics Indonesia (Badan Pusat Statistik—BPS), National Population and Family Planning Board (BKKBN), and Kementerian Kesehatan (Kemenkes—MOH), and ICF International. (2013). *Indonesia demographic and health survey (IDHS) 2012.* Jakarta, Indonesia: BPS, BKKBN, Kemenkes, and ICF International.

Thaddeus, S., & Maine, D. (1994). Too far to walk: Maternal mortality in context. *Social Science & Medicine, 38*(8), 1091–1110.

Titaley C.R, Hunter C.L, Dibley M.J, Heywood P. (2010). Why do some women still prefer traditional birth attendants and home delivery? A qualitative study on delivery care services in West Java Province, Indonesia. *BMC Pregnancy and Childbirth, 10*(43). doi: https://doi.org/10.1186/1471-2393-10-43.

United Nations (2017). The sustainable development goals report 2017. UN: New York. Retrieved March 14, 2018, from https://unstats.un.org/sdgs/files/report/2017/TheSustainableDevelopmentGoalsReport2017.pdf.

United Nations Development Programme (UNDP). (2016). *Human development report 2016.* Retrieved March 14, 2018, from http://hdr.undp.org/sites/default/files/2016_human_development_report.pdf

World Health Organization (WHO). (2015). *WHO statistical profile.* Retrieved March 14, 2018, from http://www.who.int/countries/en/

Discussion Questions

1. What are some reasons why pregnant women do not go to a health facility to give birth?
2. What is the Three Delays Model and how does it relate to this program? What are the main determinants of this delay in this community?
3. What are the benefits of community-based interventions for maternal and child health? What about the challenges?
4. What were the community engagement strategies employed in this program?

Follow-Up Reading

Castle B., Wendel M., Kelly Pryor B. N., Ingram M. (2017). Assessing community leadership: Understanding community capacity for health improvement. *Journal of Public Health Management & Practice*, *23*(4 Supp), S47–S52. doi: https://doi.org/10.1097/PHH.0000000000000587.

D'Innocenzo L., Mathieu J. E., Kukenberger M. R. (2014). A meta-analysis of different forms of shared leadership–team performance relations. *Journal of Management*, *42*(7), 1964–1991. doi: https://doi.org/10.1177/0149206314525205.

Pardosi J. F., Parr N., Muhidin S. (2017). Local government and community leaders' perspectives on child health and mortality and inequity issues in rural Eastern Indonesia. *Journal of Biosocial Science*, *49*(1), 123–146. doi: https://doi.org/10.1017/S0021932016000134.

Uneke C. J., Ezeoha A. E., Ndukwe C. D., Oyibo P. G., Onwe F. D. (2012). Enhancing leadership and governance competencies to strengthen health systems in Nigeria: Assessment of organizational human resources development. *Healthcare Policy*, *7*(3), 73–84.

Chapter 8
R U OK?: The Role of Community in Suicide Prevention

Brendan Maher

Australia: Demographics Overview
Population: 23,232,412
Life expectancy: 82.2 years

- Male: 79.8
- Female: 84.8

GNI per capita: $42,822
Literacy rate:
Total fertility rate: 1.77 children/woman
Under-five mortality rate (per 1000 live births): 4
UN HDI: 0.939
Top three causes of death

- Ischemic heart disease
- Stroke
- Alzheimer's and other forms of dementia

Suicide: A Major Public Health Concern

Globally, an estimated 800,000 people die by suicide per year, and many more attempt it. Suicide is a major public health problem that has negative social, economic, and psychological impacts on both individuals and communities (World Health Organization, 2014). In 1998, suicide constituted 1.8% of the total global disease burden; this will rise to an estimated 2.4% by 2020 (World Health Organization, 2012).

B. Maher (✉)
CEO I R U OK?, Sydney, NSW, Australia
e-mail: brendan@ruok.org.au

© Springer Nature Switzerland AG 2019
M. Withers, J. McCool (eds.), *Global Health Leadership*,
https://doi.org/10.1007/978-3-319-95633-6_8

Like in many other countries across the world, suicide is a significant public health concern in Australia. In 2017, there were 3,128 deaths by suicide with an age-specific rate of 12.7 per 100,000. This equates to an average of 8.6 deaths by suicide in Australia each day. Intentional self-harm was ranked the 13th leading cause of death in 2017, moving up from 15th position in 2016.

Deaths from intentional self-harm occur among males at a rate more than three times greater than that for females. There were 2,348 male deaths at a age-specific rate of 19.2 per 100,000. There were 780 female deaths at an age-specific rate of 6.3 per 100,000.

In 2017, 165 Aboriginal and Torres Strait Islander persons died as a result of suicide, with a standardised death rate of 25.5 deaths per 100,000 persons. When comparing intentional self-harm deaths between the Indigenous and Non-Indigenous populations, suicide accounted for a greater proportion of all Aboriginal and Torres Strait Islander deaths (5.5%) compared with deaths of Non-Indigenous Australians (2.0%) (Australian Bureau of Statistics, 2016). Intentional self-harm ranked as the 5th leading cause of death for the Aboriginal and Torres Strait Islander population.

Evidence suggests that help-seeking for suicidality is very low (Hom, Stanley, & Joiner, 2015; Luoma, Martin, & Pearson, 2002). In one study, more than one-half (55%) of people who complete suicide had no contact with a primary health-care provider in the month before suicide, and 68% had no contact with mental health services in the year before suicide (Luoma et al., 2002). In Hom et al.'s (2015) review of 12 studies among 12,000 people assessing past-year suicide ideation, plans, and/or attempts, only about 30% of this population had sought mental health services. The main barriers to seeking help include rejection of treatment or support due to hopelessness or pessimism, stigma associated with mental health problems, preference for self-management, fear of hospitalization, beliefs about lack of effective treatment, lack of perceived need for services, and structural factors, such as availability of care and lack of time or financial resources (Hom et al., 2015).

Given the magnitude of the problem, and the fact that suicide is largely preventable, more efforts are needed to prevent suicide globally. In its 2014 report, the World Health Organization (WHO) underscored the importance of the role of the community in suicide prevention. The report reinforces that social connectedness and support for an individual experiencing a crisis—partners, family members, peers, friends, and significant others—can have the most influence. Relationships are especially protective for adolescents and the elderly, who have a higher level of dependency.

Research has demonstrated that programs targeting "bystanders" or "gatekeepers" may be successful in reducing suicide attempts (Isaac et al., 2009; ORYGEN, 2010). The programs usually focus on training high school students, peers, military personnel, and clinicians, on improving recognition of the signs of suicide and depression in others and building skills on how to respond properly (Aseltine, James, Schilling, & Glanovsky, 2007; Kataoka, Stein, Nadeem, & Wong, 2007; Lipson, 2014; Michelmore & Hindley, 2012; Robinson, Green, Spittal, Templer, & Bailey, 2016; Wasserman, Hoven, Wasserman, et al., 2015; Wyman et al., 2010). The National Centre of Excellence in Youth Mental Health of Australia (ORYGEN) found that the research shows that gatekeeper training is effective at improving the knowledge, attitudes, self-efficacy, and perceived competence of gatekeepers in the short term. Studies also show promise that these programs can also influence proximal variables of suicide risk such as skill acquisition and referral behaviors of gatekeepers and adaptive norms held by young people around the acceptability of seeking help for suicide risk and perceptions of support from adults. However, few studies have examined the long-term effects, such as reduction of actual suicide attempts, of gatekeeper training programs (Isaac et al., 2015; ORYGEN, 2010).

Introduction

The History and Mission

R U OK? was founded by marketing executive Gavin Larkin in 2009 following the suicide death of his father, Barry Larkin. He hoped that by promoting the importance of open, honest communication, people would ultimately feel better supported by others, making them less vulnerable to crisis or suicide. R U OK?'s vision is "a world where all people are connected and are protected from suicide." R U OK?'s mission (as per its 2016–2019 strategic roadmap) is to "inspire and empower everyone to meaningfully connect with people around them and support anyone struggling with life." Priorities are underpinned by the following four goals:

- Knowledge—boost confidence to meaningfully connect and ask about life's ups and downs.
- Intent—nurture our sense of responsibility to regularly connect and support others.
- Impact—strengthen our sense of belonging because we know people are there for us.
- Viability—be relevant, strong, and dynamic.

R U OK? can be defined a grassroots campaign which has an enormous and growing following and uptake. It leverages significant community and corporate support. It is a primary prevention program, aimed at preventing suicide by strengthening Australia's informal community care capacity by inspiring and empowering people to meaningfully connect with and support individuals experiencing difficulties. R U OK? organizes events and provides guidance across its campaigns on how to ask, listen, encourage action (referral pathways) and check in to help prevent suicide in others.

The WHO defines informal community care as "services provided in the community but are not part of the 'formal' health and welfare system" (World Health Organization, 1999). Examples of people who can provide such services include traditional healers and professionals in other sectors such as teachers, police, village health workers, as well as laypersons in the community. Services can also be provided by community-based and nongovernmental organizations, family associations, and many more. R U OK?'s focus is to strengthen Australia's informal community care capacity to enable all Australians to have regular, meaningful conversations with family, friends, and community members to prevent suicide. The organization's main focus is strengthening suicide protective factors (specifically, connectedness and a sense of belonging), drawing on innovative and best practice expertise, evaluation, marketing, and communication principles. R U OK?'s approach is based on a growing evidence base including WHO's arguments for the importance of the role of the community in suicide prevention (World Health Organization, 2014).

Description of the Program

R U OK? began as a national mental health promotion initiative that aims to bring Australians together to prevent suicide. R U OK? targets the help-giver, not the person who is struggling. Funded partly under The Australian government Department of Health's National Suicide Prevention Program (NSPP), R U OK? promotes local community-based suicide prevention activities that will contribute to the outcomes specified in the strategic framework "Living Is For Everyone (LIFE): A framework for prevention of suicide and self-harm in Australia" (Commonwealth of Australia, 2008). The importance of informal community care was reinforced in the inaugural National Mental Health Commission of Australia's mental health report card, in which it was noted that:

> Family and friends, our local community, employers and co-workers are the foundation of support for each of us... Support from our community, GPs and other professionals play a greater role in mental health and good health overall than specialist health services or the most highly specialized care. (National Mental Health Commission, 2012)

The US academic Thomas Joiner positions "belongingness" as one of the most malleable and powerful protective factors in preventing suicidality. He has advanced the belief that if you can enhance an individual's sense of belonging, you can reduce the likelihood of suicidal behavior (Joiner, 2005). The work of Thomas Joiner and his psychosocial theory of why people die by suicide has been crucial in framing R U OK?'s mission and rationale. It is because of this framework that R U OK? seeks to enhance a person's sense of connectedness and belonging by focusing on regular meaningful conversations between family, friends, and co-workers who are struggling with life.

R U OK?: Targets

The intended beneficiaries of the R U OK? program include anyone facing difficulty or problem in life, as well as people experiencing a crisis/suicidal ideation. As seen in Fig. 8.1, it is important to note that R U OK?'s target audience is family, friends, and community members living and working alongside people at risk. In other words, R U OK? seeks to empower and activate the help-giver to provide support to the person who is struggling with life.

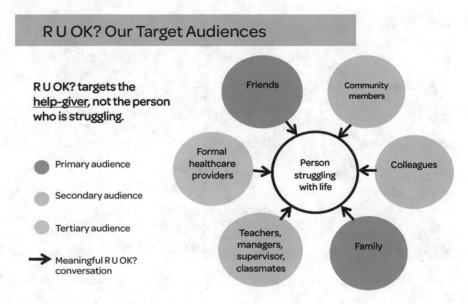

RU OK? Our Target Audiences

RU OK? targets the
help-giver, not the person
who is struggling.

● Primary audience

● Secondary audience

● Tertiary audience

➤ Meaningful RU OK?
   conversation

Friends

Community
members

Formal
healthcare
providers

Person
struggling
with life

Colleagues

Teachers,
managers,
supervisor,
classmates

Family

Fig. 8.1   R U OK?'s target audiences. Source: (R U OK website, n.d.)

Although individuals experiencing distress are not the primary targets, R U OK?
is mindful of key demographics associated with the risk of suicide, as well as the
factors which contribute to risk. As seen in Fig. 8.2, the factors that are associated
with risk of suicide can be categorized into three groups: individual level,
sociocultural level, and situational level. At the individual level, these include
mental disorders, substance abuse, social isolation, and history of trauma and abuse,
among others. At the sociocultural level, stigma and other barriers to health care
may inhibit help-seeking behavior. Exposure to suicide, including the media, is also
associated with suicide risk. At the situational level, crises such as loss of job and
stressful life events, and easy access to lethal means of suicide, increase risk.

Activities

R U OK?Day is a national day to promote regular connection in Australia which
takes place on the second Thursday in September; R U OK?Day is a national day of
action to encourage everyone to meaningfully connect with people around them and
support anyone struggling with life. R U OK?Day addresses the role of everyday
people in boosting connection (thereby reducing suicide risk); delivering messages
through traditional, digital, and social media; and linking to expert support for
conversations too big to take on alone.

R U OK?Day is complemented by yearlong campaigns and every day resources,
which are designed to meet its goal of contributing to long-term behavioral change

Individual	Socio-cultural	Situational
• Previous suicide attempt • Mental disorder • Alcohol or drug abuse • Hopelessness • Sense of isolation • Lack of social support • Aggressive tendencies • Impulsivity • History of trauma or abuse • Acute emotional distress • Major physical or chronic illnesses, including chronic pain • Family history of suicide • Neurobiological factors	• Stigma associated with help-seeking behaviour • Barriers to accessing health care, especially mental health and substance abuse treatment • Certain cultural and religious beliefs (for instance, the belief that suicide is a noble resolution of a personal dilemma) • Exposure to suicidal behaviours, including through the media, and influence of others who have died by suicide	• Job and financial losses • Relational or social losses • Easy access to lethal means • Local clusters of suicide that have a contagious influence • Stressful life events

Fig. 8.2 Depicting the framework for public health action for the prevention of suicide. Source: (WHO, 2012)

in multiple sectors, so that people feel more empowered, more confident, and more willing to have a conversation with someone they're worried about. As a health promotion campaign, R U OK? provides a number of freely available, open-source campaign resources, mostly online, designed to help people build confidence and capacity to connect and have meaningful conversations with others. It also provides opportunities and impetus for people to proactively connect. While these campaign settings target different audiences, all of R U OK?'s campaign resources provide tips and content via print, digital platforms, and broadcast media to boost the confidence and capacity of people to ask, listen without judgment, encourage action (help-seeking pathways), and check in (following-up). These campaigns include the following:

- R U OK? at Work: to boost staff's confidence to ask the question of their peers
- R U OK? Afield: for workplaces in the resource and mining sectors to remind employees to trust their instincts and dig deeper if they suspect someone is struggling with work-life balance
- R U OK? at School: for secondary students to help them champion the importance of belonging, conversations, and communities
- R U OK? Rural and Remote: targeting people living and working outside Australia's bigger towns and cities.
- R U OK? at Uni: targeting students at university and other tertiary education institutions
- R U OK? at Law: collaborative industry campaign targeting people working in the legal profession
- R U OK? in Rail: collaborative industry campaign targeting people working in the rail industry

Key Components of Leadership

R U OK? has a small staff of six and limited resources; it does not compete in a significant sense within the mental health and suicide prevention sector for government, corporate, philanthropic, and community support. However, its strong collaboration with the mental health and suicide prevention sector in Australia also provides help-seekers with a pathway to care through the promotion of appropriate services. Operating at the early continuum of care, R U OK? collaborates with and promotes mental health organizations and support services which provide expert support for people experiencing distress and suicidal thoughts or living with mental illness, as seen in Fig. 8.3.

The success of R U OK?Day, as well as its other yearlong activities, stems from true national collaboration with a multitude of stakeholders. First, it relies on strong leadership and collaboration with the mental health and suicide prevention sectors in Australia to provide help-seekers with a pathway to care through the promotion of appropriate services. For example, the organization is an active member of the Mental Health Australia and Suicide Prevention Australia. This ensures that R U OK? keeps informed of broader initiatives, policy, and reform within the mental health and suicide prevention sector and is appropriately represented as a member of the two key peak bodies in Australia. R U OK? also participates in national leadership groups including those specifically for communication leads and comprising representatives of many at-risk communities. This enables information-sharing and amplification of campaigns across organizations and sectors. R U OK?

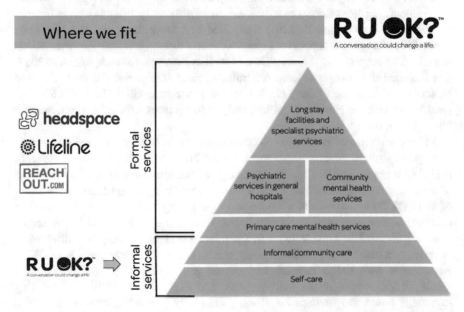

Fig. 8.3 Depicting where R U OK? fits in the mental health and suicide prevention *space*. Source: (National Mental Health Commission, 2012)

works with the mental health and suicide prevention sector to promote complementary campaigns, initiatives, and services across digital, social, and traditional media channels for both national and local organizations. R U OK? benefits from the support of the major suicide and mental health sector organizations. For example, campaign materials are designed with appropriate consultation and oversight by expert advisory committees to ensure that they are safe and designed with current best practice guidelines. These committees are a strong demonstration of a collaborative and integrated approach harnessing expertise and guidance around the development of conversation resources and evaluation. Committee members include representatives from established mental health and suicide prevention organizations in Australia. R U OK?'s partnerships with media, behavioral and evaluation experts, as well as many companies help to disseminate the message and inspire and give confidence to countless Australians to start life-changing conversations.

Second, industry-specific initiatives such as Rail R U OK?Day and R U OK? at Law provide a platform for the promotion of regular, meaningful conversations every day of the year at the workplace. Collaboration with business and industry such as hospitality, mining, transport, banking, and finance provides enhanced channels to reach significant staff and customer networks for the promotion of regular, meaningful conversations every day. Corporate partnerships with Hungry Jack's (an Australian burger chain in Australia), Virgin Mobile, Bristow Helicopters, and Sensis are enabling R U OK? to broaden its reach. With Hungry Jack's, for instance, R U OK? was able to reach over 14,000 staff with via internal communication channels and over one million weekly customers through a footprint of over 400 restaurants across Australia.

Third, R U OK? benefits from the support from all levels and parties within government, not least the Suicide Prevention Parlimentary Friends Group chaired by Julian Lesser MP and Dr Mike Kelly AM MP. Over the years, R U OK? has sucessfully engaged the support of a cross section of federal and state Parlimentarians to assist with amplyfying R U OK?Day, as well as other related campaigns. In 2017, this included direct support from Australia's Prime Minister at the time, the Hon Malcom Turnbull; the Federal Health Minister, the Hon Greg Hunt; the Shadow Health Minister, the Hon Julie Collins; and the Indigenous Affairs Minister, Senator Nigel Scullion.

Finally, with the renewed focus on consumer-centric, locally coordinated services through Australian government-commissioned Primary Health Networks (PHNs), R U OK? is committed to establishing strong and sustained dialogue with PHNs and other state government mental health agencies about current and future dovetailing of R U OK?'s activities and encouraging community participation to strengthen informal community care. The Australian government established 31 PHNs across Australia in 2015 to provide more independence on how funding was directed to improve outcomes based on community needs. While still early days, R U OK?'s engagement with PHNs includes analysis of geographical data and information about what's happening in their regions and exploring feasibility of piloting regionally based and strategic activities, particularly in remote, rural communities and indigenous groups.

Outcomes/Results

The success of R U OK? was highlighted in a peer-reviewed study of the effectiveness of the campaign (The International Journal of Mental Health Promotion, 2016). Every year it commissions an evaluation and presents findings on the Australian public's awareness and understanding of the organization. It also examines public participation in R U OK?Day activities, perceptions of the value of the campaign and supporting activity, and its perceived impact. Since the inauguration of this national day of action at Australian Parliament House in Canberra, R U OK? has become a household name. Awareness of the campaign has increased markedly over the years. A 2017 study of 2000 Australians found that an estimated 78% of Australians were aware of R U OK?, an increase of 7% from 2016. This reflects the effectiveness of the organization's marketing campaign which has largely used community-based activities, publicity, and social media, with only very limited mass media advertising. Comparisons between metropolitan and nonmetropolitan areas showed that awareness of R U OK? was slightly higher in nonmetropolitan areas. Given that rates of suicide have been found to be significantly higher in regional areas, particularly among males, this is a positive finding. The same study found that Australians continue to be highly receptive to R U OK?'s message; the organization was identified as the one that people most associate with "encouraging people to talk about things which are troubling them." In 2017, 83% made this association in the post-campaign survey (Colmar Brunton, 2017).

The vast majority of participants who had heard of R U OK? associated the campaign correctly with talking with others about what is troubling them, and a majority associated the campaign with suicide prevention. The latter finding is particularly encouraging as it provides the underlying rationale for the campaign. Of note is that this association was only slightly less than for long-established organizations in the suicide prevention area. In addition, 45% of respondents were aware that it incorporates a set of activities all year long, a slight increase from 2016 (Colmar Brunton, 2017). The awareness that R U OK? is more than an annual event helps to provide the rationale for the sustainability of its ongoing campaign activities and long-term objectives. Additionally, when asked to write down the purpose of RU OK?Day in their own words, almost all of the survey respondents referred to connecting with and supporting others.

Future Directions

R U OK? created a 2016–2019 strategic plan to more effectively complement the work of related organizations and to better leverage its unique marketing, creative, and networking skills. It is currently implementing this plan, which incorporates the continuation and further development of R U OK?Day and complementary campaigns—including a national day of action and continuation and enhancement of supporting campaigns and resources targeting high-risk groups. Within this plan, the key is the prioritization of improved resources for remote rural communities and Aboriginal and Torres Strait Islanders. In addition, the plan focuses on sharpening collaboration to reach veterans, LGBTI groups (lesbian, gay, bisexual, transgender, and/or intersex), and culturally and linguistically diverse audiences. R U OK? is also developing resources for primary school-aged children. Such resources will be freely available via its open-source approach. Another goal is to improve the relevance and accessibility of the content via social and digital channels. R U OK? also aims to continue to strengthen project reach by further leveraging mainstream media support and empowering high-profile and community ambassadors—including those from high-risk communities—to help promote key messages and activate campaigns. Finally, it will continue to seek better ways to measure impact and improve activity through better evaluation.

Conclusion

Suicide is a leading cause of death globally, requiring much more attention in terms of prevention, education, and research. "Gatekeeper" programs such as R U OK? can help reduce suicide. As a health promotion campaign, its success can be attributed to addressing an unmet need to specifically activate an individual's sense of responsibility to reach out and support someone they're worried about. R U OK? offers an exemplary and unique platform for suicide prevention awareness and community development. Through strong partnerships with media, behavioral and evaluation experts, as well as many private businesses, schools, and community groups, its works help to disseminate the message and inspire and give confidence to countless Australians to start a conversation to save a life.

References

Aseltine, R. H., James, A., Schilling, E. A., & Glanovsky, J. (2007). Evaluating the SOS suicide prevention program: A replication and extension. *BMC Public Health, 7*(1), 1.
Australian Bureau of Statistics. (2016). *Causes of death, Australia, 2016.* Retrieved February 1, 2018, from http://www.abs.gov.au/AUSSTATS/abs@.nsf/DetailsPage/3303.02016?OpenDocument.
Commonwealth of Australia. (2008). *Living Is For Everyone (LIFE) Framework (2007).* Retrieved February 2, 2018, from https://www.lifeinmindaustralia.com.au/splash-page/docs/LIFE-framework-web.pdf.
Hom, M. A., Stanley, I. H., & Joiner, T. E. (2015). Evaluating factors and interventions that influence help-seeking and mental health service utilization among suicidal individuals: A review of the literature. *Clinical Psychology Review, 40*, 28–39.
Isaac, M., Elias, B., Katz, L. Y., Belik, S. L., Deane, F. P., Enns, M. W., et al. (2009). Gatekeeper Training as a preventative intervention for suicide: A systematic review. *Canadian Journal of Psychiatry, 54*(4), 260–268.

Joiner, T. (2005). *Why people die by suicide*. London: Harvard University Press.

Kataoka, S., Stein, B. D., Nadeem, E., & Wong, M. (2007). Who gets care? Mental health service use following a school based suicide prevention program. *Journal of the American Academy of Child & Adolescent Psychiatry, 46*(10), 1341–1348.

Lipson, S. K. (2014). A comprehensive review of mental health gatekeeper-trainings for adolescents and young adults. *International Journal of Adolescent Medicine and Health, 26*(3), 309–320.

Luoma, J. B., Martin, C. E., & Pearson, J. L. (2002). Contact with mental health and primary care providers before suicide: a review of the evidence. *American Journal of Psychiatry, 159*, 909–916.

Michelmore, L., & Hindley, P. (2012). Help-seeking for suicidal thoughts and self-harm in young people: A systematic review. *Suicide and Life-threatening Behavior, 42*(5), 507–524.

National Centre for Excellence in Youth Mental Health (ORYGEN). (2010). Does gatekeeper training prevent suicide in young people? *Research bulletin issue 06*. Retrieved February 5, 2018, from file:///C:/Users/mwithers/AppData/Local/Microsoft/Windows/INetCache/Content.Outlook/UCDX43J2/Orygen_Suicide_prevention_research_bulletin.pdf.

National Mental Health Commission. (2012). A Contributing Life, the 2012 National Report Card on Mental Health and Suicide Prevention. Sydney: NMHC

R U OK?. (n.d.). Website. Retrieved February 5, 2018, from https://www.ruok.org.au/.

Robinson, J., Green, G., Spittal, M. J., Templer, K., & Bailey, E. (2016). Impact and acceptability of delivering skills based training on risk management (STORM) in Australian secondary schools. *Health Behavior and Policy Review, 3*(3), 259–268.

Wasserman, D., Hoven, C. W., Wasserman, C., et al. (2015). School-based suicide prevention programs: the SEYLE cluster-randomized, controlled trial. *The Lancet, 385*(9977), 1536–1544.

World Health Organization. (2014). *Preventing suicide: A global imperative*. Retrieved February 2, 2018, from http://apps.who.int/iris/bitstream/10665/131056/1/9789241564779_eng.pdf.

World Health Organization (WHO). (1999). *Improving health systems and services for mental health*. Retrieved February 2, 2018, from http://apps.who.int/iris/bitstream/10665/44219/1/9789241598774_eng.pdf.

World Health Organization (WHO). (2012). *Public health action for the prevention of suicide: a framework*. Retrieved February 3, 2018, from http://apps.who.int/iris/bitstream/10665/75166/1/9789241503570_eng.pdf.

Wyman, P. A., Brown, C. H., LoMurray, M., Schmeelk-Cone, K., Petrova, M., Yu, Q., et al. (2010). An outcome evaluation of the Sources of Strength suicide prevention program delivered by adolescent peer leaders in high schools. *American Journal of Public Health, 100*(9), 1653–1661.

Discussion Questions

1. Based on your own experiences and knowledge, make a list of suicide prevention campaigns that you're aware of. In your opinion, what makes these campaigns effective or ineffective?
2. How can we improve screening for mental health issues among students? If you could implement one program to target suicide prevention in the community, what would that be and why?
3. Would a campaign like R U OK? be relevant in other cultural contexts? Why or why not?
4. What are the main challenges or limitations with the gatekeeper model for suicide prevention?
5. How does stigma influence mental health care seeking behavior? Has it changed over the last few decades? What policies or programs could be instituted to reduce stigma related to suicidality?

Follow-Up Readings

R U OK? Organizational Website: http://www.ruok.org.au

Dumesnil H, Verger P. (2009). Public awareness campaigns about depression and suicide: A review. *Psychiatric Services, 60,* 1203–1213.

Van Orden K.A, Witte T.K, Cukrowicz K.C, Braithwaite S.R, Selby E.A, Joiner T.E, Jr. (2010). The interpersonal theory of suicide. *Psychological Review, 117,* 575–600.

Chapter 9
Air Pollution and Climate Change

Jonathan Samet and Alistair Woodward

United States: Demographics Overview
Population: 326,625,791
Life expectancy: 79.8 years

- Male: 77.5
- Female: 82.1

GNI per capita: $53,245
Total fertility rate: 1.87 children/woman
Under-five mortality rate (per 1000 live births): 7
UN HDI: 0.920
Top 3 causes of death:

- Ischemic heart disease
- Alzheimer's and other dementias
- Trachea, bronchus, and lung cancers

Source: CIA World Factbook (2016), UNDP Human Development Programme (2016), WHO publications (2015).

In this chapter, we describe how critical research studies can make a difference and how researchers can advance public health by fostering translation of their findings and through evidence-based advocacy. We use two examples that affect the Pacific Rim, drawing on "lessons learned" from air quality regulation in the

J. Samet
Department of Epidemiology, Office of the Dean, Colorado School of Public Health, Aurora, CO, USA

A. Woodward (✉)
Epidemiology and Biostatistics, School of Population Health, University of Auckland, Auckland, New Zealand
e-mail: a.woodward@auckland.ac.nz

© Springer Nature Switzerland AG 2019
M. Withers, J. McCool (eds.), *Global Health Leadership*,
https://doi.org/10.1007/978-3-319-95633-6_9

United States and the IPCCC. Previously, with colleagues from the Association of Pacific Rim Universities (APRU) (Wu et al., 2017), we have described approaches to air quality regulation in several Pacific Rim countries. There are different ways that leadership may be critical in advancing air quality, which include:

1. Carrying out research that provides findings that will have impact
2. Participating in the translation of the results to decision-makers in order to assure that there will be impact
3. Identifying localized problems, e.g., a polluting factory, and championing action

Background on the Issue of Climate Change

The quality of outdoor air is a common good, shared by all, and contaminated and made unhealthy by the activities of some. After decades of research, we know that air pollution can lead to premature death and to substantial morbidity and loss of well-being. While many countries have grappled with air pollution problems, two decades into the twenty-first century, some countries are experiencing still unacceptably high concentrations of air pollution, particularly some of the world's largest countries in the Asia-Pacific Rim—India and China (Cohen et al., 2017). In contrast, most high-income countries have greatly improved air quality through regulatory initiatives and also the transfer of polluting industries to other countries.

Air pollution control is evidence-based and driven to a great extent by the findings of epidemiological studies but supported by complementary work involving animal and human exposure studies and laboratory studies on the ways that air pollution causes injury. The epidemiological studies have identified the adverse effects of air pollution and also described how risks for these effects vary along the range of exposures experienced in the population. In some countries and particularly the United States, there are well-worked-out frameworks for using scientific evidence in setting air quality standards. In contrast, some low-income countries lack such frameworks, and some do not even have the most basic measures of air quality, such as concentrations of airborne particulate matter.

One widely recognized air pollution threat is climate change, resulting from our exceedance of the atmosphere's capacity to contend with the rate of greenhouse gas emissions. This problem requires coordinated global action. Here, we focus on the role of the Intergovernmental Panel on Climate Change (the IPCC).

Evidence and Air Quality Standards

Air pollution has long been a problem, exacerbated by the industrial revolution, fossil fuel combustion for heating and electric power generation, and motor vehicle emissions. In-depth research on air pollution and health was sparked by the 1952

London fog, which led to at least 10,000 excess deaths as particle levels likely reached perhaps 100 times typical levels in urban environments in high-income countries today (Bates, 2002). The findings of the initial research were clear—air pollution increases mortality; adversely affects children and others who are susceptible, e.g., older persons and those with heart and lung diseases; and contributes to general ill health. The findings were also sufficient to motivate action to control air pollution through regulatory actions in many countries.

In the ensuing decades, research on the health consequences of air pollution has continued, using increasingly sophisticated methods. The list of adverse consequences of air pollution has continued to lengthen, and the levels at which effects are observed has moved lower and lower. The most recent studies show adverse effects at routine concentrations in cities in high-income countries including the United States, Canada, and various European countries (Beelen et al., 2014; Di, Dai, et al., 2017; Di, Wang, et al., 2017).

Systems have been developed for integrating and evaluating the evidence in support of evidence-based air quality regulation. One model is that used by the US Environmental Protection Agency (EPA) (Fig. 9.1) for developing the National Ambient Air Quality Standards or NAAQS. The process begins with evidence and moves through steps including evidence evaluation, consideration of exposures and risks, and the elaboration of policy options. This US-based approach has evolved over the almost 50 years since the Clean Air Act was passed in 1970. Under that act, the EPA administrator is called on to set NAAQS that protect public health with "an adequate margin of safety."

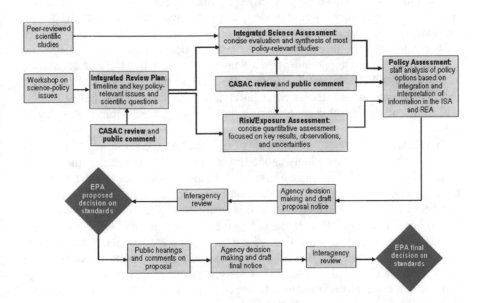

Fig. 9.1 Process for reviewing National Ambient Air Quality Standards. Source: (US Environmental Protection Agency, 2009)

Case Studies

Airborne Particulate Matter and Mortality

Airborne particulate matter (PM) refers to the complex mixture of particles that can be found in outdoor (and indoor) air; the particles differ in their sources, composition, and toxicity. Depending on the location, the source mix includes motor vehicles, power generation from combustion, trash burning, biomass fuel combustion, industries, and nature—e.g., blowing sand, pollens, and sea salts. Airborne particles are classified by their size, which has bearing on the sites that they reach in the lung when inhaled. The most widely used indicator at present is $PM_{2.5}$, referring to particles that have an aerodynamic diameter less than 2.5 μm. Such particles come largely from man's activities, and they are small enough to reach the lung's small airways and the alveoli or air sacs. Particles in the $PM_{2.5}$ size range have been linked to adverse effects on the health of children, worsening of heart and lung diseases, and risk for premature mortality.

This case study focuses on the emergence of the scientific evidence on PM and premature mortality, the ensuing controversy, and the efforts by various industries to derail action based on scientific evidence. It illustrates the potential power of scientific evidence and the need for resilience on the part of researchers when their studies are attacked.

This case study begins, largely in the United States, in the early 1990s several decades after the Clean Air Act had resulted in improved air quality and to a level that was thought perhaps to be protective of public health. A series of publications provided evidence contrary to this view. The emerging research came from what are termed "daily time-series" studies: studies in which the basic data involve daily counts of death, often grouped by cause and age, concentrations of PM and other pollutants, and temperature (Bell, Samet, & Dominici, 2004; Kelsall, Samet, Zeger, & Xu, 1997; Schwartz & Dockery, 1992). The analytical approach estimates the associations of PM and/or other pollutants with the daily mortality counts, while controlling for other time-varying factors, such as temperature and day of week.

In the early 1990s, there was a trickle of such studies, soon followed by a torrent as this methodology was widely applied to routinely collected environmental and vital statistics data. The surprise of the initial time-series studies was their positive findings: PM was associated with increased mortality on a day-to-day basis in a number of locations (Philadelphia and others; for example, Utah Valley and Santa Clara). Much criticism followed concerning the validity of the data and the analytical methods used, while another line of criticism suggested that the associations observed might reflect only a small advancement of the time of death, perhaps only a few days, which would not constitute an adverse effect. This potential form of life shortening was initially referred to as "harvesting" and later "mortality displacement" with the implication that the lives of ill people were only slightly and perhaps mercifully shortened. Some statistical approaches were used to estimate the extent of life shortening, but the results were uncertain. The concerns about the data and the methods were set aside through a project requested by the US Congress that replicated the original studies (Samet, Zeger, & Berhane, 1995). This approach of replication by an independent group has proved to be valuable for addressing controversies around pivotal data sets.

In 1993, the first study on the longer-term associations of air pollution with mortality was reported with findings suggesting that the associations observed in the daily studies did not reflect mortality displacement alone, i.e., that air pollution shortened the lifespan. This publication in the *New England Journal of Medicine* was based on the Harvard Six Cities Study of air pollution (Dockery et al., 1993). In the study, participants from six US cities, selected to cover a range of air pollution exposure, were followed and their deaths tracked. The results were striking: those living in the most polluted city had a 26% overall increased risk of dying compared with those in the least polluted city, taking into account other factors including tobacco smoking and socioeconomic status. Predictably, many points of criticism were raised, given the implications of the findings. However, in 1995, the findings of the first report were replicated, by a group including some of the same investigators, using another cohort (longitudinal) study: the American Cancer Society's Cancer Prevention Study (CPS) II (Pope III et al., 1995).

A tsunami of criticism followed, given the regulatory and public health implications of the findings and the timing of the reports, coinciding with the review of evidence for possible revision of the US NAAQS for PM. Together, the findings of the many time-series studies and the emerging evidence were sufficiently compelling to warrant a more stringent PM standard. Beyond the usual comments about methodological problems by stakeholders and their surrogates, a call mounted for release of the cohort study data, termed "secret," for analysis by industry stakeholder groups. Underlying the call were claims that the analyses and reporting were selective and biased toward positive findings. The investigators at Harvard (particularly Douglas Dockery and Joel Schwartz, along with Arden Pope at Brigham Young University) did not release the data citing correctly their commitments to maintaining privacy and confidentiality, as guaranteed with informed consent.

Again, at the request of Congress as with the time-series studies, a reanalysis of the data from the two pivotal studies was carried out with funding from the Health Effects Institute, a nonprofit jointly funded by the US EPA and vehicle manufacturers (Samet et al., 1995). A robust and transparent mechanism was established for this purpose with an oversight committee representing multiple stakeholders. The original findings were replicated, and the analyses extended to set aside an array of issues.

Still, however, the controversy continues, even as findings of more studies have been reported and certainty has increased that exposure over the longer term to PM pollution increases risk for dying. The Republican-led House Committee on Science, Space, and Technology has continued to push for release of the data, even issuing a subpoena (a request under the law) that the EPA provides the data to the committee; the Agency does not have the data. In the misnamed HONEST Act, the Committee proposed that the EPA could not use research findings in its regulatory and other actions unless data access was possible. To date, the HONEST Act has not become law; it has been resisted by individual scientists and some professional organizations, recognizing its impact on evidence-based regulation.

This case study will be continuing as research continues. The same tactics persist with more recent reports based on nationwide studies using the databases of the US Medicare system, which covers health care for the elderly (Di, Dai, et al., 2017; Di, Wang, et al., 2017).

The 2015 Paris Climate Agreement and the Intergovernmental Panel on Climate Change

Climate change is a significant global health challenge. Much is now known about why it has occurred and its consequences, as a result of research by a global community of scientists; sensing the significance of the problem, many have vigorously participated in the dissemination and translation of their work. That effort is the focus of this case study.

Climate change has resulted from disruption of planetary systems, and the impacts are now being felt in every population. The increase in atmospheric greenhouse gas levels has occurred more quickly than at any time in the last 700,000 years—consequences worldwide include rising temperatures, more extreme patterns of rainfall, accelerated sea level rise, and a 60% increase in ocean acidity. Climate change operates on a very longtime scale (changes in atmospheric CO_2 persist for centuries, for instance), and thus the process of change is essentially irreversible. There are tipping points, thresholds beyond which environmental change shifts track and it is difficult to predict outcomes. The effects on health occur largely through the multiplication of existing risks—more heat waves, more intense droughts, and greater pressure on food supplies and safe water resources. Consequently, the effects are felt most acutely by groups that are presently marginal and disadvantaged and that already experience poor health. However, no population is immune, due to the force and reach of the changes in the world's climate system occurring now. The devastating effects of extreme storms in the United States in 2017 are evidence of this.

Climate change is a global health issue in another sense—dealing with the problem requires a worldwide response. No government by itself can control the emissions of greenhouse gases and degradations in land use that are responsible for global warming. Atmospheric CO_2 does not respect national borders, and the effects, such as on food supplies and displaced populations, reverberate around the globe.

The United Nations Framework Convention on Climate Change (UNFCCC) was signed in 1992 at the Earth Summit in Rio de Janeiro. This convention provided a framework for international cooperation to combat climate change by limiting the rise in temperatures and coping, as far as possible, with the anticipated impacts. The Convention aims to "avoid dangerous climate change" and to support efforts to minimize harm. Under the Convention, the signatories agreed to meet annually, as the so-called Conference of the Parties.

In December 2015, representatives of 196 governments met in Paris at a very special meeting. For the first time, there was consensus about steps that should be taken to deal with climate change. The document adopted at the meeting spells out targets and charts a collective course of action. It was ratified more quickly than expected, and now (early 2018) all but one of the UNFCCC governments has formally signed up. The Paris Agreement is the world's first comprehensive climate agreement.

It is certainly ambitious. At Paris, governments agreed to limit warming to well below 2 °C above pre-industrial temperature and to advance efforts to hold warming to less than 1.5 °. (Global average temperature is presently close to 1 ° above the nineteenth-century benchmark for "pre-industrial.")

The agreement acknowledges the urgency of the challenges—emissions "must peak as soon as possible." In addition to controlling emissions, the agreement explicitly recognizes the importance of adaptation and the need for the global community to fund protection in the most vulnerable countries.

There are targets—which are not imposed "top-down" but are based on the Intended Nationally Determined Contributions (INDCs) that countries brought to Paris. Each state decided its commitment in advance of the meeting. The real weight in the Paris Agreement lies in the sections to do with review and reporting. Signatories agreed to monitor and report on progress against the INDCs, with a hard review at 5 years. The 5-year check is intended to act as a "ratchet" mechanism, to extend and strengthen national actions.

There are limitations and weaknesses in the Agreement. The INDCs are not sufficient. Even if fully implemented, it is projected that by 2100 warming will reach 2.6–3.1 °C (Rogelj et al., 2016). The national targets carry no legal force, and there are no secure financial systems to ensure the need for adaptation is met. And the current president of the United States, the country with the second biggest emission footprint and the most technologically developed economy, has signaled US withdrawal.

But the Paris Climate Agreement stands nevertheless as a high point in international efforts to respond to climate change. How did it happen? An important factor was the way that the 2015 meeting was organized—described as "a triumph of climate diplomacy" (Obergassel, Arens, Hermwille, & Kreibich, 2015). Success factors include the careful preparations made long before delegates arrived in Paris and especially assiduous courting of heads of state. National leaders, including Presidents Barack Obama and Xi Jinping, attended the meeting, and importantly, they were present at the beginning of the talks (rather than making a fly-in appearance at the end), to help generate momentum and set directions. The organizers took pains to make the process as open, participatory, and transparent as possible. The indaba style of negotiating was adopted, which focuses on specific problems or "red lines" and the solutions to these problems, and does not permit parties to repeatedly state and defend broad positions. Potential critics of the agreement were drawn into the process and, in many cases, given responsible positions in the negotiations. And the French government ensured that this all happened in what was called "an impeccable environment," where practicalities of large and demanding meetings were managed with aplomb, reducing wherever possible the stresses on the delegates.

The Agreement is not just an example of fine diplomacy, however. The agreement was built on a foundation of scientific understanding. Here we look at one specific source of technical advice on climate change, the Intergovernmental Panel on Climate Change (IPCC), explore its contribution to the Paris Agreement, and focus on the role of individual scientists who took leading positions on climate change.

The IPCC was established in 1988 by the UN Environment Program and the World Meteorological Office as a scientific body charged with advising governments on all aspects of climate change. The members of the Panel are technically the states that are signed up to the UNFCC. But the work is done by scientists appointed by the Panel and guided by a standing body, the Bureau of the IPCC. Outputs from the IPCC include special reports (recent examples include publications on renewable energy, land use and terrestrial ecosystems, and extreme events) and the regular assessment reports. The latter are prepared on roughly 6-year cycles and include reports on physical systems, impacts of climate change and adaptation, and mitigation.

In this case study, we will examine the most recent assessment report, the fifth (AR5), which was published in 2013/2014, and will focus particularly on the findings relevant to human health.

First is some background on how the assessment reports are prepared. These are large-scale endeavors—considered together, the IPCC reports probably represent the largest scientific assessment exercise ever. There were 310 coordinating and lead authors responsible for the second volume in AR5, that on impacts and adaptation. Orchestrating the work of this large group falls on the shoulders of the co-chairs of each working group. Typically, these individuals are chosen to balance input from high-income and developing countries, and in AR5, Working Group 2 was headed by Dr. Chris Field (from Stanford University in the United States) and Dr. Vicente Barros from Argentina.

Aspects of the IPCC process distinguish its outputs from other scientific publications. One is the intensity of peer review, more intense and prolonged than what scientists usually experience. For example, the authors of the human health chapter in AR5 received 1009 reviewer comments on the second order draft; there were four iterations of review and response in all.

Another important feature is the significant role of member states in determining the scope of the reports and approving the final output. IPCC authors work independently: government input occurs as part of the peer review process. However, the member states scrutinize and sign off the final product, adding a challenging and potentially onerous aspect to the work of the co-chairs. They are responsible to lead the member states' delegates through the summary for policymakers, the section of the report that contains the key findings. Before the report is adopted, every word and phrase of the summary must be agreed upon, by the full meeting. United Nations rules apply here— the resolution must be unanimous. Line by line, the delegates are led through the 30–40-page summary. The co-chairs must be in command of the science, since the content can be questioned at any point, but they must also pay scrupulous attention to process.

The plenary meetings that sign off on IPCC reports are essentially international negotiations, although the subject is a distillation of scientific advice. Field and Barros, like other co-chairs, had to manage national posturing, advocacy for particular interests, and, in some instances, straightforward obstructionism. Like many international negotiations, the plenary meetings may include prolonged and exhausting sessions, especially toward the end of allotted time, as what took place in the fifth assessment. The co-chairs required extraordinary stamina, patience, and a portfolio of diplomatic skills.

We summarize here the major findings of AR5 that are relevant to health—full details are available on the IPCC website or in Woodward et al. Woodward et al. (2014). First, there is unequivocal warming of the climate system underway, and many changes are unprecedented. Human influence on these changes is unmistakable. Human health is sensitive in many respects to climate and weather, and the imprint of climate change is now apparent, particularly through occurrence of damaging extreme events such as heat waves. Attribution science has advanced sufficiently to now permit confident statements about the likelihood that events such as the Russian heat waves and fires of 2010 are due to human-induced climate change.

AR5 focused particularly on the projected impacts in this century but did not restrict its discussion to this time window. The report pointed out that many young children born recently can expect to live past 2100, and this is the generation that will experience so-called "long-term" impacts in the next century. Looking so far ahead is difficult, but projections of the high emissions scenario for greenhouse gases, RCP8.5, underline the severity of unmitigated climate change. The health chapter warned that in the early 2100s, "the capacity of the human body to thermo-regulate may be exceeded on a regular basis, particularly during manual labor" … "raising doubt about the habitability of some areas." In other words, adaptation is necessary and important, but is not sufficient on its own, since continuing climate change will run up against hardwired limits.

Throughout the impacts and adaptation report, the importance of rates of change was stressed. The speed of climate change and the variability of exposures such as temperatures and precipitation are risk factors in their own right. It is not just the

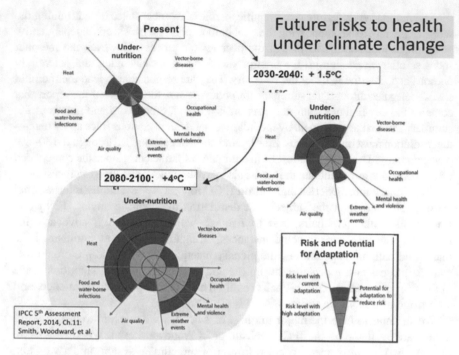

Fig. 9.2 Future risks to health. Source: (IPCC, 2014)

magnitude of warming but the rapidity of onset and the uncertainty of its course of change matter, in terms of coping capacities. The speed of warming and its unprecedented progress are significant warning signs.

With an eye to the decisions that governments need to make, AR5 attempted to distinguish between the risks of "moderate" warming (1.5–2 °) from those associated with higher levels (typically around 4 ° by 2100). The health chapter estimated how much of these future impacts may be managed by high-level adaptation (Fig. 9.2.). Moderate warming was projected to threaten health through many pathways, including heat, undernutrition, and food and waterborne infections, but there may be capacity, in many areas, to buffer the adverse effects by well-funded adaptation. These include better agriculture practices, greater investment in food safety and secure water supplies, and heat wave planning. Health problems resulting from disruptions to the global food supply were highlighted in the high warming scenario, along with the risks of violence and disorder. In this instance, it is uncertain whether these risks could be substantially managed by better services or improvements in production.

The report concluded that the most effective adaptation measures for health in the near term were basic public health measures in settings where health was already under threat. However, it was emphasized that further climate-specific measures (such as early warning systems for extreme weather) would be required, for all populations, as climate change proceeds.

Are the findings of AR5 reflected in the conditions of the 2015 Paris Climate Agreement? To a large extent, they are. The ambitious targets adopted in Paris are consistent with the conclusions of the assessment report that climate change is already underway, that its adverse effects are now seen, and that the future risks, while uncertain, are serious. The IPCC report emphasized the importance of adaptation in the immediate future, given the climate change in progress from historical emissions. The IPCC described the differential impacts and the greater vulnerability of resource-poor and disadvantaged communities. It also sketched out differences between a low warming trajectory and the effects of a trajectory that matches in many respects "business as usual" in climate policy (i.e., only light-handed restrictions on the use of fossil fuels). The risks of "business as usual," including the crossing of significant thresholds in coping capacity, make it urgent that net emissions are reduced as quickly as possible.

While the IPCC reports are produced by teams, individuals play a vital part in leadership. Key are the chair of the IPCC (Rajendra Pachauri in AR5—an industrial engineer from India) and the co-chairs of the working groups. Their roles include the initial high-level negotiations with member states over the content and balance of the reports, and guiding the selection of writing teams, which must include the necessary technical expertise, and at the same time balance geographical and disciplinary input. Shepherding the reports through the final plenary sessions, as described above, is the final step in the politico-scientific process. Leadership positions in the IPCC are high profile, and individuals in these posts are liable to criticism from all quarters. Whether the IPCC is thought to be too timid, too ambitious, too slow, or irresponsibly hasty, the chairs and co-chairs may be held to account. Robert Watson, chair of the IPCC until 2002, was ousted from the job following pressure from the United States. Over the year preceding, the Republican administration, under President George W. Bush, had been heavily lobbied by fossil fuel interests for a change in IPCC leadership, given what was seen as a strong anti-oil and gas bias in the second and third assessment reports (IPCC, 2014).

There are examples of other climate change scientists, many contributors to the IPCC, who have faced controversy because of their work. Michael Mann, a paleoclimate specialist, was widely criticized in the early 2000s over the so-called hockey stick controversy, a reconstruction of early Earth climate. Mann's work has been confirmed by subsequent research. Phil Jones, an atmospheric scientist from the United Kingdom who took part in the IPCC assessments in 2001 and 2007, was pilloried in the popular press after a large number of emails were stolen from his workplace, the University of East Anglia in 2009, and selected correspondence was leaked. The purpose was to discredit the Climate Research Unit that he led. Although a subsequent inquiry by a committee of the House of Commons found there was no case for Jones to answer, he never returned to the position he held when the email leak occurred.

It remains to be seen whether the Paris Climate Agreement will be sustained and whether it will lead to substantial improvements in greenhouse emissions, land use practices, and other drivers of climate change. But it should be noted that what was agreed upon in Paris reflects, in essential matters, what was contained in the most recent report of the body commissioned by governments to provide technical advice. Here is an example of a contribution made by scientists to resolution of a fraught, complex, and terribly important global health problem, achieved sometimes at a significant personal cost.

Lessons Learned from the Case Studies

Airborne Particulate Matter and Mortality

- Evidence on the environment and public health have important consequences, as in the example of the studies of airborne PM.
- With powerful implications for regulation, research findings will inevitably be scrutinized and criticized, and the skills and integrity of researchers may be questioned.
- In the example of the studies of PM, the investigators and their institutions stood firm, rebutting criticisms and not releasing data and thus adhering to commitments made to participants. Their approach represents a useful example for others placed into similar situations.
- Reanalysis proved to be a robust mechanism for affirming the credibility of findings.

The 2015 Paris Climate Agreement and the Intergovernmental Panel on Climate Change

- Big problems require "big science," and synthesis of evidence may require large, interdisciplinary teams.
- Achieving a globally uniform response to climate change has proved challenging. The framework convention has been a framework for response.
- Antagonistic stakeholders can delay progress.
- As with PM, researchers may be threatened.

Key Components of Leadership

These two case studies illustrate that the foundation for change is solid scientific evidence. Researchers can lead change by doing research that counts. They have a role in translational activities, like the IPCC. Most critically, they may need to engage in evidence-based advocacy, favoring policies supported by the evidence and have a certain degree of "toughness" to deal with stakeholder tactics.

Conclusion

Outdoor air quality has improved in many countries as a result of better understanding of the nature of the hazard, the relation between exposures and disease, and the effectiveness of interventions. Health professionals have initiated and conducted critical pieces of research, have taken the lead in communication of the findings, and have been active in evidence-based advocacy. This applies also to climate change, in which CO_2 and other greenhouse pollutants have a global impact, and emissions continue to rise year on year. The response must similarly be on a global scale; progress depends on international research collaborations and energetic and skillful leadership at the science-policy interface.

References

Bates, D. V. (2002). A half century later: Recollections of the London fog. *Environmental Health Perspectives, 110*(12), A735.

Beelen, R., Raaschou-Nielsen, O., Stafoggia, M., Andersen, Z. J., Weinmayr, G., Hoffmann, B., et al. (2014). Effects of long-term exposure to air pollution on natural-cause mortality: An analysis of 22 European cohorts within the multicentre ESCAPE project. *Lancet, 383*(9919), 785–795. https://doi.org/10.1016/S0140-6736(13)62158-3

Bell, M. L., Samet, J. M., & Dominici, F. (2004). Time-series studies of particulate matter. *Annual Review of Public Health, 25*, 247–280. https://doi.org/10.1146/annurev.publhealth.25.102802.124329

Central Intelligence Agency (CIA) (2016). *CIA world Factbook*. Retrieved March 20, 2018, from https://www.cia.gov/library/publications/the-world-factbook/.

Cohen, A. J., Brauer, M., Burnett, R., Anderson, H. R., Frostad, J., Estep, K., et al. (2017). Estimates and 25-year trends of the global burden of disease attributable to ambient air pollution: An analysis of data from the global burden of diseases study 2015. *Lancet, 389*(10082), 1907–1918. https://doi.org/10.1016/s0140-6736(17)30505-6

Di, Q., Dai, L., Wang, Y., Zanobetti, A., Choirat, C., Schwartz, J., et al. (2017). Association of short-term exposure to air pollution with mortality in older adults. *JAMA, 318*(24), 2446–2456. https://doi.org/10.1001/jama.2017.17923

Di, Q., Wang, Y., Zanobetti, A., Wang, Y., Koutrakis, P., Choirat, C., et al. (2017). Air pollution and mortality in the Medicare population. *New England Journal of Medicine, 376*(26), 2513–2522. https://doi.org/10.1056/NEJMoa1702747

Dockery, D. W., Pope III, C. A., Xu, X., Spengler, J. D., Ware, J. H., Fay, M. E., et al. (1993). An association between air pollution and mortality in six U.S. cities. *New England Journal of Medicine, 329*(24), 1753–1759.

IPCC (2014). *Climate change 2014: Impacts, adaptation, and vulnerability. A contribution of working group II to the fifth assessment report of the intergovernmental panel on climate change* [Field, C.B., V.R. Barros, D.J. Dokken, K.J. Mach, M.D. Mastrandrea, T.E. Bilir, M. Chatterjee, K.L. Ebi, Y.O. Estrada, R.C. Genova, B. Girma, E.S. Kissel, A.N. Levy, S. MacCracken,P.R. Mastrandrea, and L.L. White (eds.)]. Geneva: World Meteorological Organization, 190 pp.

Kelsall, J. E., Samet, J. M., Zeger, S. L., & Xu, J. (1997). Air pollution and mortality in Philadelphia, 1974-1988. *American Journal of Epidemiology, 146*(9), 750–762.

Obergassel, W., Arens, C., Hermwille, L., & Kreibich, N. (2015). Phoenix from the ashes: An analysis of the Paris agreement to the United Nations Framework Convention on climate change; part 1. *Environmental Law and Management, 27*(6), 243–262.

Pope III, C. A., Thun, M. J., Namboodiri, M. M., Dockery, D. W., Evans, J. S., Speizer, F. E., et al. (1995). Particulate air pollution as a predictor of mortality in a prospective study of U.S. adults. *American Journal of Respiratory and Critical Care Medicine, 151*(3), 669–674.

Rogelj, J., Elzen den, M., Höhne, N., Fransen, T., Fekete, H., Winkler, H., et al. (2016). Paris agreement climate proposals need a boost to keep warming well below 2 °C. *Nature, 2534*(7609), 631–639.

Samet, J.M., Zeger, S., Berhane, K. (1995). *Particulate air pollution and daily mortality: Replication and validation of selected studies*. Cambridge, MA: Retrieved March 30, 2018, from https://www.healtheffects.org/system/files/Special-Report-PEEP-Phase-IA-with-corrected-page-35.pdf.

Schwartz, J., & Dockery, D. (1992). Increased mortality in Philadelphia associated with daily air pollution concentrations. *The American Review of Respiratory Disease, 145*, 600–604.

U.S. Environmental Protection Agency. (2009). *Process for reviewing national ambient air quality standards*. Retrieved March 30, 2018, from https://www3.epa.gov/ttn/naaqs/pdfs/NAAQSReviewProcessMemo52109.pdf.

United Nations Development Programme (UNDP) (2016). *Human development report 2016*. Retrieved March 20, 2018, from http://hdr.undp.org/sites/default/files/2016_human_development_report.pdf.

Woodward, A., Smith, K., Campbell-Lendrum, D., Chadee, D., Honda, Y., Liu, Q., et al. (2014). Climate change and health: On the latest IPCC report. *Lancet, 383*(9924), 1185–1189.

World Health Organization (WHO). (2015). *WHO statistical profile*. Retrieved March 20, 2018, from http://www.who.int/countries/en/.

Wu, C., Woodward, A., Li, Y. R., Kan, H., Balasubramanian, R., Latif, M., et al. (2017). Regulation of fine particulate matter ($PM_{2.5}$) in the Pacific rim: Perspectives from the APRU Global Health program. *Air Quality, Atmosphere and Health, 10*, 1039–1049. https://doi.org/10.1007/s11869-017-0492-x

Discussion Questions

1. What are some general pathways for using scientific evidence to develop policy? How can individual researchers lead for change?
2. What has been the role of air pollution researchers in improving air quality?
3. What should researchers do when their research and their integrity is questioned?
4. How has the translation of research findings to policymakers and the public been important in terms of air pollution and climate change policies?

Follow-Up Reading

Cohen, A., Brauer, M., Burnett, R., Anderson, H., Frostad, J., Estep, K., Forouzanfar, M. (2017). Estimates and 25-year trends of the global burden of disease attributable to ambient air pollution: An analysis of data from the Global Burden of Diseases Study 2015. *The Lancet, 389*(10082), 1907–1918.

Watts, N., Amann, M., Ayeb-Karlsson, S., Belesova, K., Bouley, T., Boykoff, M., Costello, A. (2018). The Lancet Countdown on health and climate change: From 25 years of inaction to a global transformation for public health. *The Lancet, 391*(10120), 581–630.

Woodward, A., Smith, K., Campbell-Lendrum, D., Chadee, D., Honda, Y., Liu, Q., Haines, A. (2014). Climate change and health: On the latest IPCC report. *The Lancet, 383*(9924), 1185–1189.

Wu, C., Woodward, A., Li, Y., Kan, H., Balasubramanian, R., Latif, M., Samet, J. (2017). Regulation of fine particulate matter (PM2.5) in the Pacific Rim: Perspectives from the APRU Global Health Program. *Air Quality, Atmosphere & Health*, 10(9), 1039–1049.

Chapter 10
Preventing Sexual Assault on College Campuses in the United States

Mellissa Withers

> **United States: Demographics Overview**
> *Population*: 326,625,791
> *Life expectancy:* 79.8 years
>
> - Male: 77.5
> - Female: 82.1
>
> *GNI per capita: $53,245*
> *Total fertility rate: 1.87 children/woman*
> *Under-five mortality rate (per 1000 live births): 7*
> *UN HDI: 0.909*
> *Top three causes of death*
>
> - Ischemic heart disease
> - Alzheimer's and other dementias
> - Trachea, bronchus, and lung cancers
>
> Source: CIA World Factbook (2016), UNDP Human Development Programme (2016), WHO publications (2015)

Sexual assault is recognized as a serious public health problem on college campuses in the United States (US). Sexual assault is any type of sexual contact or behavior that occurs without explicit consent of the recipient, including touching, oral sex, penetration, or attempted rape, whether by physical force or threat of force or because an individual was incapacitated and unable to provide consent (US DOJ, 2017). In 2017, almost ten million females and 7.6 million males attended college in an undergraduate program in the United States (NCES, 2017). Female college

M. Withers (✉)
Keck School of Medicine, USC Institute for Global Health, Los Angeles, CA, USA
e-mail: mwithers@usc.edu

© Springer Nature Switzerland AG 2019
M. Withers, J. McCool (eds.), *Global Health Leadership*,
https://doi.org/10.1007/978-3-319-95633-6_10

students have notably high rates of sexual assault (Black et al., 2011; CDC, 2014). While sexual assaults can occur anytime throughout a lifetime, the vast majority of first sexual assaults are experienced before age 25 years (Breiding et al., 2011). Women ages 18–24 years who are college students are three times more likely than women in general to experience sexual violence (US DOJ, 2014). Being a victim of dating violence or sexual assault, especially rape, can significantly negatively impact students' mental and physical health and is associated with depression, anxiety, and substance abuse, as well as poor academic performance and school dropout (Amar & Gennaro, 2005; Baker et al., 2016; Conoscenti, McCauley, Kilpatrick, Resnick, & Ruggiero, 2007; Jordan, Combs, & Smith, 2014; Kaukinen, 2014; Lindquist et al., 2013; Lombardi, 2010; Perez-Pena, 2013; Zinzow et al., 2011).

Introduction

The US government has taken steps to respond to this form of violence against women over the last three decades through several key laws and programs. This chapter will delineate the scope of sexual assault among female college students and outline the recent and historical steps that have been taken to address the problem. While stakeholders such as victims' rights groups have been critical of the response of the government, academic institutions, and law enforcement, this case analyzes the government's leadership role in mandating increased reporting and investigation of these crimes by colleges. Although sexual assault happens to males and can also be perpetrated by females, this chapter focuses on those perpetrated by a male against a female, which are by far the most common type of assault (Krebs, Lindquist, Warner, Fisher, & Martin, 2007). The term "college" refers to any academic institutions of higher education, such as two- or four-year colleges or universities.

Numerous studies have documented the high prevalence of sexual assault among college students in the United States, showing that about one in five women experience sexual assault while in college (Cantor et al., 2015; Krebs et al., 2016). The Campus Climate Survey on Sexual Assault and Sexual Misconduct included more than 150,000 students across 27 universities and is one of the largest surveys on this topic. The incidence of sexual assault or misconduct among female undergraduates was 23.1% (Cantor et al., 2015). The 2015 Washington-Post Kaiser Family Foundation surveyed 1053 people aged 17–26 years who were undergraduates at a four year academic institution at some point since 2011, representing more than 500 institutions. Twenty-five percent of women reported unwanted sexual incidents in college, with 20% reporting sexual assault (Anderson & Clement, 2015).

Most sexual assaults of college students are perpetrated by a fellow student, current or ex dating partners, or friends (Conoscenti et al., 2007; Fisher, Cullen, & Turner, 2000; Lindquist et al., 2013). Sexual assaults most often occur off campus rather than on campus (Fisher et al., 2000). The first year of college is the most dangerous in terms of risk of sexual assault (Cantor et al., 2015; Kimble, Neacsiu, Flack, & Horner, 2008). For example, in one study, 16.9% of females reported sexual assault during their first year of college (Cantor et al., 2015). More than 50% of college sexual assaults occur in the first few months of the academic year (Kimble et al., 2008), demonstrating a heightened vulnerability among new students. This may be related, in part, to the use of alcohol; research has shown that alcohol and drug use significantly increase the risk of sexual assault, especially among first year students. Most sexual assaults of college students occur after the victim is incapacitated, either due to alcohol or drugs, which are usually voluntarily consumed by the victim but sometimes given to her without her knowledge (Cantor et al., 2015). Lindquist et al.'s (2013) study among 3951 undergraduate women at four colleges found that almost one-half of incapacitated sexual assaults happened at a party, usually on a Friday or Saturday night. About 65% of incapacitated sexual assault victims were drunk (compared to only 12% of physically forced sexual assaults), and perpetrators reportedly used alcohol or drugs prior to the assault in 72.3% of these cases.

Available data on sexual assault likely underestimate the true scope of the problem because sexual assault is difficult to measure and is severely underreported (Fisher, Daigle, Cullen, & Turner, 2003; Lindquist et al., 2013). Research shows that the vast majority of sexual assaults of college students are not reported to colleges or to law enforcement (Cantor et al., 2015; Fisher et al., 2000; Krebs et al., 2016; Zinzow et al., 2011). Krebs et al. (2016) found that only 7% of female college students who experienced sexual assault had reported it to the college. The most common reason for not reporting was that it was not considered serious enough; other reasons included embarrassment; shame, because it would be too emotionally difficult; and doubts that anything would be done about it (Cantor et al., 2015). Conoscenti et al. (2007) found that only 12% of college women had reported their sexual assault to law enforcement. Barriers to reporting included not wanting others to know about the rape, fear of retaliation, perception of insufficient evidence, uncertainty about whether a crime was committed or harm was intended, and uncertainty about whether the incident was "serious enough" (Conoscenti et al., 2007). Furthermore, research has shown that sexual assaults involving the consumption of alcohol or drugs are less likely to be reported to campus officials (Zinzow et al., 2011).

Key Policies and Programs

Title IX of the US 1972 Education Amendments prohibits discrimination on the basis of sex in academic institutions that receive federal funding (the vast majority of institutions) (US DOJ, 2015). When this law passed, it was not intended to relate to sexual violence. However, in response to court cases beginning in the 1980s in which students sued colleges for mishandling sexual assault reports, the US Supreme Court ruled that sexual harassment and sexual assault are forms of sex discrimination which can negatively impact victims' educational environment (Wilson, 2014). Under Title IX, academic institutions are legally required to respond to and remedy hostile educational environments, regardless of whether the case is pursued in criminal courts. Academic institutions also have an obligation to punish sexual misconduct with educational sanctions, as with other types of misconduct (Edwards, 2015). They must also adopt and publish grievance procedures providing for the prompt and equitable resolution of sexual assault complaints, investigate reports of sexual assault, and take swift action to prevent their recurrence. They must have a designated Title IX representative and provide students with information on programs aimed at preventing sexual assault and on procedures to report sexual assault. Survivors must be provided with information on support and services. Complaints of non-compliance can be filed with the Department of Education or against the institution itself (CHE, 2017). Institutions that fail to comply risk losing federal funding.

In response to increased awareness regarding the disturbingly high rates of college sexual assault, since the passage of Title IX, the US government has instituted several new federal laws and programs, notably the Clery Act, the Violence Against Women Act, the "Dear Colleague" letter, and the Campus Sexual Violence Elimination Act.

The Clery Act

The Jeanne Clery Disclosure of Campus Security Policy and Campus Crime Statistics Act ("Clery Act"), signed in 1990, requires all colleges that participate in federal financial aid programs to collect and disclose information about crime on and near their campuses. The law is named after Jeanne Clery, a 19-year-old Lehigh University student who was raped and murdered in her campus residence hall in 1986. Her murder sparked a backlash against unreported crime on campuses (Clery Center, 2016).

The Violence Against Women Act

The Violence Against Women Act (VAWA) was signed in 1994 by President Clinton with overwhelming support by both parties in Congress. It has been subsequently reauthorized several times. It was developed through extensive grassroots efforts, with strong support from sexual assault advocates, victim services, law enforcement, and prosecutors. Stakeholders such as victim advocates, law enforcement, prosecutors, judges, probation and corrections officials, health care professionals, and religious leaders at both state and local levels have worked together in a coordinated effort to address domestic and sexual violence (Legal Momentum, 2017). It provided over US$1.6 billion, as well as other resources, for the investigation and prosecution of violent crimes against women, imposed automatic mandatory restitution on those convicted, and allowed civil suits in cases not prosecuted in criminal courts. The Office on Violence Against Women and the White House Task Force to Protect Students from Sexual Assault were also established as a result.

Dear Colleague Letter of 2011

The "Dear Colleague" letter relating to sexual assault among college students was issued by the Office for Civil Rights (OCR) in 2011 as a powerful reminder of the requirements to prevent sexual harassment and investigate complaints of incidents taking place on and off campus. Although there were no new regulations, the letter provided specific guidelines on what may have previously been misunderstood. The letter reiterated that institutions must adopt and publish procedures for prompt and equitable resolution of sex discrimination complaints, recommending a 60-day limit for investigations. It also reminded institutions that the burden of proof required for colleges to take action is less than in criminal courts (US OCR, 2011).

Campus Sexual Violence Elimination (SaVE) Act

In 2013, the Campus Sexual Violence Elimination (SaVE) Act was signed as an amendment to the Clery Act to increase transparency about the scope of sexual violence on campus and guarantee victims' rights. It requires that colleges educate students, faculty, and staff on the prevention of rape, domestic violence, dating violence, sexual assault, and stalking. It increases standards of campus response and disciplinary proceedings (NSVRC, 2015). In addition to sexual assault, colleges must now report statistics for domestic violence, dating violence, and stalking occurring on campus, on public property within and adjacent to campus, and at noncampus properties like off-campus student housing and remote classrooms. Data on these incidents must now be collected from multiple sources, including student housing managers, athletic coaches, campus police or security, and local law enforcement. Institutions must publish procedures to afford all students and employees who report an incident of sexual violence specific rights whether or not they pursue a formal complaint (Clery Act, 2016).

Challenges

While these efforts were lauded as important steps in addressing the problem, many have criticized enforcement of them, arguing that the responsibility of documenting and investigating such crimes is largely left to individual colleges that have an interest in concealing them. Sexual assault survivors and advocate groups have called for a more concerted and coordinated approach, including better investigation of such crimes, more accountability of colleges, and for adequate punishment of perpetrators. Allegations have been made that some colleges have deliberately ignored reports of sexual assault involving student-athletes. In January 2016, Florida State settled a lawsuit for almost US$1 million by a former student who alleged that the university obstructed the investigation of a sexual assault involving a football player. In 2016, former Vanderbilt University football player Brandon Vandenburg was found guilty of the rape of an unconscious woman in his dorm room (Wade, 2017). Perhaps the most scandalous case, in 2016 Stanford University student Brock Turner was convicted of sexually assaulting a woman who was unconscious on campus. He ultimately spent only three months in a county jail for the crime, sparking widespread outrage (Fanz, 2016). A 2009 investigation on campus sexual assault by the Center for Public Integrity found that students deemed "responsible" for alleged sexual assaults can face little or no consequence for their acts while victims' lives are frequently dramatically negatively impacted (Lombardi, 2010).

In what has been called a snowball effect, these cases sparked activism among survivors, who banded together to file complaints with the government against their colleges for mishandling sexual assault complaints (Perez-Pena, 2013). For example, in January 2013, students at the University of North Carolina, Chapel Hill, Yale University, Amherst College, and others who had similar experiences filed a Title IX complaint with the US Department of Education (Perez-Pena, 2013). In 2013, prominent attorney Gloria Allred, representing eight students at Occidental College, linked those students to students who had filed similar complaints from several other institutions, including University of Southern California, University of California at Berkeley, Swarthmore College, and Dartmouth College. These high-profile groups capitalized on the media attention they garnered to heighten public awareness of the problem, hoping to demonstrate that it was not isolated to select colleges. This informal national network of survivors allowed survivors to share experiences and rally for changes at their own colleges and nationwide. Several formal advocacy organizations have also been established by survivors and activists to put pressure on colleges and the federal government to respond to what they call a national epidemic. These include End Rape on Campus, Know Your IX, and the Student Coalition Against Rape (SCAR). Such advocacy efforts have made a difference. In response, the government has reminded academic institutions of their responsibilities and has provided support to help colleges improve their response to sexual violence on campus.

Reports of sexual assault by colleges have surged dramatically in the past 15 years. A 205% increase was seen – with 2200 cases in 2001 increasing to 6700 cases in 2014. During the same period, all other reported on-campus crimes decreased (CHE, 2017). As of 2016, more than 200 institutions are under federal investigation for mishandling sexual assault and harassment cases, an increase of more than 300% since 2014 (CHE, 2017). Yet, concerns remain that colleges continue to violate rules in handling sexual violence cases. One analysis revealed that 89% of the approximately 11,000 colleges that provided annual crime data in 2015 reported zero incidences of rape. In 2015, only about 9% of campuses disclosed incidents of domestic violence, around 10% disclosed incidents of dating violence, and about 13% disclosed stalking. Furthermore, 89% of institutions reported *zero* rape in 2015 (AAUW, 2017). This underscores a serious problem in the way data are being collected, as sexual assaults are clearly not being reported to campus authorities. The Clery Act only requires that crimes that occur on or adjacent to campuses are reported. Krebs et al. (2016) compared data from the Campus Climate Survey Validation Study to Clery Act data in 2015 for nine institutions. Of the 2380 total rapes that occurred among students, only 60 fit the criteria for reporting under the Clery Act, and only 40 of them were actually reported. While 770 rapes had occurred on campus, only 160 of them were reported to authorities, who would have then been required to report them under the Clery Act.

Although progress has clearly been made in reporting and investigating campus sexual assaults, momentum may stall with President Trump. Just a few months after he assumed office, Education Secretary Betsy DeVos announced new Title IX guidelines, which she said were devised to better protect the rights of the accused. Secretary DeVos implied that a large proportion of sexual assault accusations are false and said that those accused of sexual assault needed more protection from the assumption of guilt. The changes included removing the 60-day deadline for investigations, allowing accused to appeal, and implying that institutions must only address sexual misconduct that is "severe, persistent or pervasive" (Tatum, 2017). Organizations such as the Foundation for Individual Rights in Education (FIRE) and Title IX For All, a men's advocacy group, have argued that the investigation process has favored accusers and unfairly penalizes the accused. Over 200 lawsuits have been filed against universities for violating the rights of students accused of sexual assault (Title IX, 2017). However, a 2015 White House report on rape found that only 2–10% of sexual assault reports are false (White House Council on Women and Girls, 2014). President Trump himself has been accused of sexual assault by at least 19 women (Ford, 2017).

In 2017, rampant sexual misconduct in many sectors came to light. In January 2017, the Women's March was a worldwide protest which united more than 2.5 million people on women's issues including violence against women and violations of women's rights. Later that year, several famous and powerful male figures lost their jobs due to sexual misconduct, including TV personalities Bill O'Reilly and Charlie Rose. Then, high-profile movie mogul Harvey Weinstein was exposed as a serial predator of young actresses, triggering a domino effect. US Senator Al Franken, actor Kevin Spacey, comedian Louis CK, and former host of the popular morning show Today Matt Lauer, among others, were also fired after reports of inappropriate sexual behavior. By the end of 2017, more than 60 prominent men were suspended, fired, or forced to resign because of allegations of sexual harassment and assault, some occurring many years before. This inspired a global social medial campaign, the #MeToo Movement, which called upon women to publicly acknowledge their experiences of sexual misconduct to demonstrate the pervasiveness of the problem. On Facebook, the hashtag was used by more than 4.7 million people in 12 million posts during the first 24 h (France, 2017; Santiago & Criss, 2017). The "Silence Breakers", women who accused powerful men of sexual misconduct, were named Time Magazine's "person of the year" (Presutti, 2017). The Movement galvanized support around the world, sparking a similar trend in which politicians, media stars, and other powerful figures lost their jobs as a result of sexual misconduct. In January 2018, Time's Up, a movement against sexual harassment, was founded to help fight sexual violence and harassment in the workplace through lobbying and providing funding for victims to get legal help if they can't afford it. It lobbies for legislation that creates financial consequences for companies that regularly tolerate harassment without action. The Movement took center stage during the Golden Globe Awards, where most women wore black as a sign of solidarity and to protest sexual abuse (The Associated Press, 2018).

Conclusions

While these are positive steps in addressing violence against women, more must be done to ensure that all college students are provided with safe learning environments. In addition to better enforcement of current policies already in place, several additional measures by colleges are recommended, including more education, better support systems for students who report sexual assaults, and more accountability and transparency in investigating these events. The shockingly high number of colleges that report zero sexual assaults implies that students are not comfortable reporting such incidents to school officials. The vast majority of colleges have clearly not implemented effective procedures to encourage reporting and to provide support to sexual assault survivors. Prevention programs in the community are needed to help address the problem of violence against women at a societal level.

References

Amar, A. F., & Gennaro, S. (2005). Dating violence in college women: Associated physical injury, health care usage, and mental health symptoms. *Nursing Research, 54*, 235–242.

American Association of University Women (AAUW). (2017). *89 Percent of Colleges Reported Zero Incidents of Rape in 2015*. Retrieved January 5, 2018, from http://www.aauw.org/article/clery-act-data-analysis-20171/4.

Anderson, N., & Clement, C. (2015). One in five college women say they were violated. *The Washington Post*. Retrieved January 9, 2018, from http://www.washingtonpost.com/sf/local/2015/06/12/1-in-5-women-say-they-were-violated/?utm_term=.ed97841819a1.

Baker, M. R., Frazier, P. A., Greeg, C., Paulsen, J. A., Howard, K., Meredith, L. N., et al. (2016). Sexual victimization history predicts academic performance in college women. *Journal of Counseling Psychology, 63*(3), 685–692.

Black, M.C., Basile, K.C., Breiding, M.J., Smith, S.G., Walters, M.L., Merrick, M.T., et al. (2011). *The national intimate partner and sexual violence survey: 2010 summary report*. Retrieved January 19, 2018, from http://www.cdc.gov/violenceprevention/pdf/nisvs_report2010-a.pdf.

Breiding, M.J., Smith, S.G., Basile K.C., Walters, M.L., Chen, J., & Merrick, M.T. (2011). *Prevalence and characteristics of sexual violence, stalking, and intimate partner violence victimization—National intimate partner and sexual violence survey, United States, 2011*. Atlanta, GA: Centers for Disease Control and Prevention. Retrieved from March 14, 2018, https://www.cdc.gov/mmwr/preview/mmwrhtml/ss6308a1.htm.

Cantor, D., Fisher, B., Chibnall, S., Townsend, R., Lee, H., Bruce, C., et al. (2015). *American Association of University Women Climate Survey on Sexual Assault and Sexual Misconduct*. Retrieved January 7, 2018, from https://www.aau.edu/sites/default/files/AAU-Files/Key-Issues/Campus-Safety/AAU-Campus-Climate-Survey-FINAL-10-20-17.pdf.

Centers for Disease Control and Prevention (CDC). (2014). *Preventing sexual violence on college campuses: Lessons from research and practice*. Retrieved January 7, 2018, from https://www.notalone.gov/schools/.

Central Intelligence Agency (CIA). (2016). *CIA World Factbook*. Retrieved from https://www.cia.gov/library/publications/the-world-factbook/

Chronicle of Higher Education (CHE). (2017). Sexual assault investigator tracker. Retrieved January 10, 2018 https://projects.chronicle.com/titleix/

Clery Center. (2016). *The campus sexual violence elimination act*. Retrieved January 9, 2018, from http://www.cleryact.info/campus-save-act.html.

Conoscenti, L.M., McCauley, J., Kilpatrick, D.G., Resnick, H.S., & Ruggiero, K.J. (2007). *Drug-facilitated, incapacitated, and forcible rape: A national study. National Criminal Justice Reference Service*. Retrieved January 9, 2018, from https://www.ncjrs.gov/pdffiles1/nij/grants/219181.pdf.

Edwards, S. (2015). The case in favor of OCR's tougher title IX policies: Pushing back against the pushback. *Duke Journal of Gender Law & Policy, 23*(1), 121–144.

Fanz, A. (2016). *Outrage over 6-month sentence for Brock Turner in Stanford rape case. CNN*. Retrieved January 7, 2018, from http://www.cnn.com/2016/06/06/us/sexual-assault-brock-turner-stanford/index.html

Fisher, B.S., Cullen, F.T., & Turner, M.G. (2000). *The sexual victimization of college women*. US Department of Justice, Office of Justice Programs, Bureau of Justice Statistics. Retrieved March 14, 2018, from https://www.ncjrs.gov/pdffiles1/nij/182369.pdf.

Fisher, B. S., Daigle, L. E., Cullen, F. T., & Turner, M. G. (2003). Reporting sexual victimization to the police and others: Results from a national-level study of college women. *Criminal Justice and Behavior, 30*(1), 6–38.

Ford, M. (2017). *The 19 women that have accused President Trump of sexual misconduct. The Atlantic*. Retrieved January 17, 2018, from https://www.theatlantic.com/politics/archive/2017/12/what-about-the-19-women-who-accused-trump/547724/

France, L.R. (2017). *#MeToo: Social media flooded with personal stories of assault*. Retrieved January 12, 2018, from http://www.cnn.com/2017/10/15/entertainment/me-too-twitter-alyssa-milano/index.html

Jordan, C. E., Combs, J. L., & Smith, G. T. (2014). An exploration of sexual victimization and academic performance among college women. *Trauma, Violence, & Abuse, 15*(3), 191–200.

Kaukinen, C. (2014). Dating violence among college students: The risk and protective factors (link is external). *Trauma, Violence, & Abuse, 15*(4), 283–296.

Kimble, M., Neacsiu, A., Flack, W., & Horner, J. (2008). Risk of unwanted sex for college women: Evidence for a red zone. *Journal of American College Health, 56*(3), 331–337.

Krebs, C. P., Lindquist, C. H., Berzofsky, M., Shook-SA, B., Peterson, K., Planty, M., et al. (2016). *Campus climate survey validation study: Final technical report*. Washington, D.C.: U.S. Department of Justice, Bureau of Justice Statistics.

Krebs, C. P., Lindquist, C. H., Warner, T. D., Fisher, B. S., & Martin, S. L. (2007). *The campus sexual assault (CSA) study*. Washington, DC: National Institute of Justice, U.S. Department of Justice.

Legal Momentum. (2017). *History of the Violence Against Women Act*. Retrieved January 7, 2018, from https://www.legalmomentum.org/history-vawa

Lindquist, C. H., Barrick, K., Krebs, C., Crosby, C. M., Lockard, A. J., & Sanders-Phillips, K. (2013). The context and consequences of sexual assault among undergraduate women at historically black colleges and universities (HBCUs). *Journal of Interpersonal Violence, 28*(1), 2437–2461.

Lombardi, K. (2010). *A lack of consequences for sexual assault. The Center for Public Integrity*. Retrieved January 8, 2018, from https://www.publicintegrity.org/2010/02/24/4360/lack-consequences-sexual-assault

National Center for Education Statistics (NCES). (2017). *Indicators of school crime and safety 2016*. Retrieved January 8, 2018, from https://nces.ed.gov/fastfacts/display.asp?id=372.

National Sexual Violence Resource Center (NSVRC). (2015). *Fact sheet: Campus sexual assault*. Retrieved January 9, 2018, from http://www.nsvrc.org/sites/default/files/publications_nsvrc_factsheet_media-packet_campus-sexual-assault.pdf.

Perez-Pena, R. (2013). College groups connect to fight sexual assault. *The New York Times*. Retrieved January 4, 2018, from http://www.nytimes.com/2013/03/20/education/activists-at-colleges-network-to-fight-sexual-assault.html.

Presutti, C. (2017). *2017 marked a sea change in attitudes towards sexual misconduct*. Retrieved January 12, 2018, from https://www.voanews.com/a/sexual-harassment-charges-in-2017/4178023.html.

Santiago, C., & Criss, D. (2017). *An activist, a little girl, and the heartbreaking origin of 'me too.'* Retrieved January 12, 2018, from http://www.cnn.com/2017/10/17/us/me-too-tarana-burke-origin-trnd/index.html.

Tatum, S. (2017). *Devos announces review of Obama-era sexual assault guidance*. CNN. Retrieved January 9, 2018, from http://www.cnn.com/2017/09/07/politics/betsy-devos-education-department-title-ix/index.html.

The Associated Press. (2018). *Winfrey says 'time is up" for abusive men in Globes speech*. Retrieved January 12, 2018, from https://www.nytimes.com/aponline/2018/01/07/us/ap-us-golden-globes-oprah.html.

Title IX For All. (2017*). Milestone 200 lawsuits alleging due process and related claims*. Retrieved January 9, 2018, from http://www.titleixforall.com/milestone-200-lawsuits-alleging-due-process-and-related-claims/.

United Nations Development Programme (UNDP). (2016). *Human Development Report 2016*. Retrieved March 14, 2018, from http://hdr.undp.org/sites/default/files/2016_human_development_report.pdf.

US Department of Justice. (2015). *Title IX of the education amendments of 1972*. Retrieved January 9, 2018, from https://www.justice.gov/crt/title-ix-education-amendments-1972.

US Department of Justice, Office of Justice Programs, Bureau of Justice Statistics. (2014) *Rape and sexual victimization among college-aged females, 1995-2013*.

US Department of Justice, Office on Violence Against Women. (2017). *Sexual assault*. Retrieved January 6, 2018, from https://www.justice.gov/ovw/sexual-assault#sa.

US Office of Civil Rights (OCR). (2011). *Dear colleague letter from assistant secretary for civil rights Russlynn Ali*. Retrieved January 10, 2018, from http://www2.ed.gov/about/offices/list/ocr/letters/colleague-201104.html.

Wade, L. (2017). 'Frat stars and athletes- those are the only ones that matter': Here's the dark truth of campus hookup culture. *Business Insider*. Retrieved January 7, 2018, from http://www.businessinsider.com/the-dark-truth-about-rape-on-college-campus-2017-3.

White House Council on Women and Girls. (2014). *Rape and sexual assault: A renewed call to action*. Retrieved January 9, 2018, from https://obamawhitehouse.archives.gov/sites/default/files/docs/sexual_assault_report_1-21-14.pdf.

Wilson, R. (2014). Why colleges are on the hook for sexual assault. *The Chronicle*. Retrieved January 9, 2018, from https://www.chronicle.com/article/Why-Colleges-Are-on-the-Hook/146943.

World Health Organization (WHO). (2015). *WHO statistical profile*. Retrieved March 14, 2018, from http://www.who.int/countries/en/.

Zinzow, H. M., Amstadter, A. B., McCauley, J. L., Ruggiero, K. L., Resnick, H. S., & Kilpatrick, D. G. (2011). Self-rated health in relation to rape and mental health disorders in a national sample of college women. *Journal of American College Health, 59*(7), 588–594.

Discussion Questions

1. Why do you think first year students are particularly vulnerable to sexual assault?
2. What are some unique challenges that female college students who have experienced sexual assault may face in accessing help? And how can colleges better respond to support these students?
3. How much of the responsibility for preventing and responding to sexual assault should be assumed by the federal government versus the individual college?
4. What are some specific interventions that colleges could take that might be effective in preventing sexual assault on college campuses?
5. How might the recent movements to expose sexual misconduct in other sectors influence sexual assault on college campuses?

Follow–Up Reading

Centers for Disease Control and Prevention (CDC). (2016). Sexual assault on campus. strategies for prevention. https://www.notalone.gov/schools/.

DeGue, S. (2014). A systematic review of primary prevention strategies for sexual violence perpetration. *Aggression and Violent Behavior, 19*(4), 346–362.

Krebs, C. P., Lindquist, C. H., Berzofsky, M., Shook-S. A. B., Peterson, K., Planty, M., Langon, L., & Stroop, J. (2016). *Campus climate survey validation study: Final technical report.* Washington, D.C.: U.S. Department of Justice, Bureau of Justice Statistics.

McMahon, S., Valle, L.A., Holt, M.K., Massetti, G.M., Matjasko, L., & Tharp, A. T. (2011). *Changing perceptions of sexual violence over time.* National Online Resource Center on Violence Against Women. http://www.ncdsv.org/images/Vawnet_ChangingPerceptionsOf SexualViolenceOverTime_10-2011.pdf

Chapter 11
National Cancer Control in Korea

Jae Kwan Jun and Keun-Young Yoo

Republic of Korea: Demographics Overview
Population: 51,181,299*Life expectancy*: 82.4 years

- Male: 79.3
- Female: 85.8

GNI per capita: $34,541
Total fertility rate: 1.26 children/woman
Under-five mortality rate: 4
UN HDI: 0.901
Top 3 causes of death

- Stroke
- Ischemic heart disease
- Self-harm

Sources: CIA World Factbook (2016), UNDP Human Development Report (2016), WHO Statistical Profile (2015)

Cancer has been the leading cause of death in Korea since 1983 (Korean Statistical Information Service, 2017). Reducing the cancer burden at the national level is likely to receive increasing attention in the near future. Due to Korea's rapidly aging population, a major increase in cancer incidence is expected in the next couple of decades. Additionally, risk factors associated with cancer incidence

J. K. Jun (✉)
National Cancer Control Institute, National Cancer Center, Goyang, Republic of Korea
e-mail: jkjun@ncc.re.kr

K.-Y. Yoo
Department of Preventive Medicine, Seoul National University College of Medicine,
Seoul, Republic of Korea

Armed Forces Capital Hospital, Seongnam, Republic of Korea

© Springer Nature Switzerland AG 2019
M. Withers, J. McCool (eds.), *Global Health Leadership*,
https://doi.org/10.1007/978-3-319-95633-6_11

and cancer-related mortality, including tobacco use, alcohol consumption, obesity, and physical inactivity, remain major concerns (Ma et al., 2017).

In 2015, a total of 217,057 (112,882 males and 104,175 females) cases were newly diagnosed with cancer. The overall crude incident rates (CR) were 444.9 and 410.3 per 100,000 for males and females, respectively, and age-standardized incidence rates (ASR) were 302.2 and 255.5 per 100,000 for males and females, respectively. Among males, the five leading primary cancer sites were stomach (CR 79.2, ASR 52.7), lung (CR 66.0, ASR 43.7), colon and rectum (CR 63.8, ASR 42.6), liver (CR 47.5, ASR 31.4), and prostate (CR 38.6, ASR 25.6) (Fig. 11.1). Among females, the most common cancers were thyroid (CR 97.0, ASR 69.8), breast (CR 72.1, ASR 47.7), colon and rectum (CR 42.5, ASR 23.0), stomach (CR 38.5, ASR 21.4), and lung (CR 28.7, ASR 14.9).

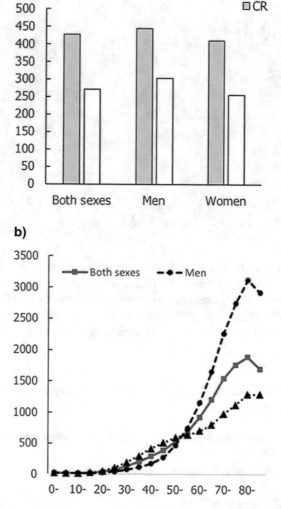

Fig. 11.1 Cancer incidence by gender (**a**) and age (**b**) in Korea, 2014. Notes: *CR* crude rate, *ASR age-standardized incidence rate* using the Segi's world standard population. Source: Jung et al. (2017)

Introduction

The Korean government's first cancer control policy was developed by the Ministry of Health and Welfare (MOHW), when in 1989 it highlighted the need to establish a national center dedicated to cancer and began formulating a plan to establish such a center. In 1996, the government initiated a comprehensive "10-Year Plan for Cancer Control" (Yoo, 2007). In response to the public need to create a national institution devoted to research, clinical care, and education and training related to cancer, the Korean National Cancer Center (NCC) was founded in March 2000 under the NCC Act. Since then, the NCC, in close cooperation with MOHW, has played a key role in formulating and implementing national cancer control programs, such as the development of the cancer prevention programs and national cancer screening guidelines (Lee, Shin, & Kim, 2001). The NCC consists of three main divisions: the Research Institute, Hospital, and National Cancer Control Institute (NCCI). The Research Institute of the NCC pursues excellence in cancer research by concentrating on translational research that produces promising results, which can be applied directly to cancer patients and people at risk of developing cancer. Staffed by high-caliber medical personnel, the most up-to-date medical equipment, and an optimal operation system, the 500-bed NCC Hospital provides cancer patients with the best available clinical care services (National Cancer Center, 2017). In 2005, the NCCI was set up to assist the government in implementing the evidence-based national cancer control policies effectively. The Cancer Control Act, a legal framework for controlling cancer in Korea legislated in 2003, authorizes the NOHW to formulate and implement cancer control programs and promote international collaboration. In early 2006, the comprehensive second-term cancer control plan (2006–2015) was forged to strengthen the cancer control efforts at the government level within the following framework (Fig. 11.2) (Han, Choi, Park, Moor, Park et al., 2011).

Description of the Programs

Anti-smoking Program

The National Health Promotion Act of 1995 stipulates that all public facilities must designate smoking and non-smoking areas. The Act has restricted the installation of cigarette vending machines and prohibits selling cigarettes to minors under age 19. In 2001, the government initiated an anti-smoking programs with the aim of reducing the adult male and adolescent male smoking rates to 29.0% and 9.0%, respectively, by 2020 (Korea Health Promotion Institute, 2017). In 2015, smoking prevalence was 39.3% for men and 5.5% for women (Korea Centers for Disease Control & Prevention, 2017c). In 2017, 6.3% of Korean adolescents (9.5% among males and 3.1% among females) said that they have smoked one or more days in the

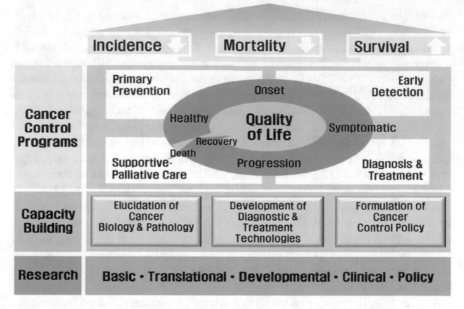

Significant Reduction of Cancer Burden

Incidence   Mortality   Survival

Cancer Control Programs	Primary Prevention	Onset	Early Detection
Healthy Quality of Life Symptomatic	Recovery	Death
Supportive-Palliative Care	Progression	Diagnosis & Treatment

| Capacity Building | Elucidation of Cancer Biology & Pathology | Development of Diagnostic & Treatment Technologies | Formulation of Cancer Control Policy |

| Research | Basic · Translational · Developmental · Clinical · Policy |

Fig. 11.2 Scheme of the Korean Government for cancer control. Source: Han et al. (2011)

previous 30 days (Korea Centers for Disease Control & Prevention, 2017b). The prevalence of e-cigarette use was 4.2% for males and 0.4% for females in 2016 (Korea Centers for Disease Control & Prevention, 2017a). The government will revise the National Health Promotion Act for the successful implementation of the anti-smoking programs if the 2020 targets are not met.

Several government ministries and agencies are involved in the tobacco control efforts. The recommendations set forth by the World Health Organization and the Framework Convention on Tobacco Control have been used as guidelines. For example, the Ministry of National Defense provides anti-smoking education for military personnel and prohibited the sale of tax-free cigarettes in 2009. The MOHW launched the Quitline program in 2006: Quitline is operated by the NCC with consignment from the MOHW that sponsors Quitline with funds raised by cigarette taxes (Yun et al., 2016). It provides private counseling to help people who want to quit. There are 243 public health centers that are running smoking cessation clinics, offering counseling and pharmacotherapy (NRT and bupropion) free of charge to help people who want to quit (Oh et al., 2013). In Korea, since 2015, 17 local tobacco control centers are providing tailored smoking cessation services. Smoking cessation services that are provided by local tobacco control center include smoking cessation camps and proactive smoking cessation services, such as counseling from trained cessation counselors. The target population of local tobacco control centers are smokers who want to quit but face difficulties in using smoking cessation clinics in public health centers because of barriers such as time limitations and prejudice toward smokers. The MOHW has implemented, or will implement by 2020, the following additional policies: (a) limit cigarette advertisements in domestic periodical magazines to 30 advertisements a year; (b) obligate tobacco industries to label ingredients such as nicotine, tar, and other major carcinogens; (c) obligate tobacco companies to display the warning, "Smoking causes lung cancer and other diseases and is especially hazardous to the health of adolescents and pregnant women" on cigarette packets with a pictogram; (d) expand medical examinations of smoking-related diseases; (e) prohibit promoting tobacco sales in local government organization; and (f) expand public anti-smoking campaigns.

The Ministry of Education has also agreed to crack down on the sale of cigarettes to minors in collaboration with other government agencies. The Ministry of the Interior and Safety will strengthen the crackdown on the sale of cigarettes to minors, failure to designate smoking and non-smoking areas in buildings, and smoking in non-smoking areas.

HBV Vaccination for Hepatitis B Control and Liver Cancer Prevention

The hepatitis B virus (HBV) is a well-known risk factor for chronic liver disease and liver cancer (Choi, Han, Kim, & Lim, 2017). Korea was previously classified as an area of high endemicity for the HBV, but plasma-derived HBV vaccines, introduced in 1983, have reduced the risk to intermediate endemicity. In Korea, the first national HBV vaccination program began in 1985 for newborns whose mothers were HBV carriers. The program was extended to all health insurance beneficiaries and school-aged children in 1988 and all newborns in 1991. In 1995, HBV vaccination was integrated into the routine childhood immunization schedule. In 2015, the prevalence of HBsAg among Koreans aged 10 years and over was 3.7% in males and 2.9% in females, with a lower prevalence (less than 1.0%) in those under 20 years according to the 2015 National Health and Nutrition Survey (Park et al., 2015).

Nationwide Cancer Registration

The cancer registry is an essential part of national cancer control. In Korea, a hospital-based nationwide cancer registry, the Korea Central Cancer Registry (KCCR), was established by the MOHW in 1980. The headquarters, originally located in the National Medical Center during 1983–2000, later moved to the NCC in 2000. The number of participating hospitals and registered malignancies has increased over time, and, as of 2017, more than 180 hospitals were currently participating. KCCR data covers 97.8% of new cancer cases in Korea (Jung et al.,

2017). To accurately measure the national cancer incidence and to construct a useful database for conducting basic cancer research and treatment planning, population-based regional cancer registries were established in 1995 with financial and technical support from the KCCR. Statistics of eight regional and nationwide cancer incidences from 1999 to 2002 were officially included in the report *Cancer Incidence in Five Continents*, Volume IX, which was published online in November 2007 (International Agency for Research on Cancer, 2017), demonstrating that Korea now produces high-quality cancer-related statistics.

Enhancing Public Awareness of Cancer Control and Prevention Through Education, Training, and Campaigns

Since 2001, the NCC has offered education and training for health professionals, enabling them to promote and activate the cancer control program in their regions. These programs have been especially effective in improving public awareness about the importance of the primary cancer prevention, early detection, and palliative care activities. The NCC, along with MOHW, announced the Ten Codes for Cancer Prevention in 2006 (Table 11.1), which are guidelines the public should follow in their everyday lives, such as smoking cessation, healthy diets, regular exercise, and routine medical checkups for early detection of cancer (Kye, Park, Oh, Park et al., 2015).

The National Cancer Information Center (NCIC) was launched in 2005 to provide the comprehensive cancer information services for cancer patients, their families, the general public, and cancer professionals. Its mission is to give up-to-date, evidence-based information, as well as practical advice and support to relieve people of the fear or uncertainty of cancer (Kye, Yoo, Lee, Jun et al. 2015). The service is provided via telephone, website, and publications. The NCIC website (www.cancer.go.kr) currently receives more than 100,000 hits per month (Kye, Lee, Yoo, Oh, Jun et al., 2017). This web portal includes in-depth information on common cancers, FAQ, national cancer statistics, various kinds of educational materials, and terminologies about cancer. Moreover, NCIC also offers the most up-to-date cancer research information for cancer professionals.

National Cancer Screening Program

After the National Cancer Screening Guidelines were developed in 2001, the Korean Government embarked on the National Cancer Screening Program (NCSP) for stomach, breast, and cervical cancer in 2002, adding liver cancer in 2003 and colorectal cancer in 2004. The NCSP covers all Korean men and women and gives recommendations on age at first screening: cervix and uteri (age 20), stomach,

Table 11.1 Ten Codes for Cancer Preventions

Symbol	Code
	Don't smoke and avoid smoke-filled environments
	Consume sufficient amounts of fruits and vegetables and balance your diet with a wide range of healthy foods
	Limit your salt intake from all sources, and avoid burnt or charred foods
	Don't drink alcoholic beverages, not even less than one or two drinks per day, for cancer prevention
	Engage in at least 30 min of regular, moderate physical activity on most days of the week
	Maintain your body weight within a healthy range

(continued)

Table 11.1 (continued)

Symbol	Code
	Ensure vaccination against HBV and HPV following the vaccination schedule
	Engage in safe sexual behavior to avoid sexually transmitted disease
	Follow all health and safety instructions at work places; aim to prevent exposure to know cancer-causing agents
	Undergo routine checkups following the cancer screening programs

Source: Yoo (2007)

breast, and liver (age 40), and colon and rectum (age 50). In 2002, the NCSP began free screening for Medical Aid Program (MAP) beneficiaries and NHI beneficiaries within the lowest 20% income bracket and then extended the service to the lowest 50% income bracket in 2005. NHI beneficiaries in the upper 50% income bracket can receive screening with only a 10% out-of-pocket payment (Kim Jun, Choi, Lee, Park et al., 2011).

Participation rates for the NCSP increased annually since 2002. In 2002, screening rates were 4.3% for stomach cancer, 3.3% for liver cancer, 4.1% for colorectal cancer, 4.6% for breast cancer, and 0.9% for cervical cancer. In 2012, participation rates for stomach, liver, colorectal, breast, and cervical cancer screening were 47.3, 25.0, 39.5, 51.9, and 40.9%, respectively (Suh et al., 2017) (Table 11.2).

Table 11.2 Current protocol of the National Cancer Screening Program in Korea

Cancer	Target population	Interval	Test or procedure
Stomach	40 and over (men and women)	Every 2 years	Upper endoscopy or upper gastrointestinal (UGI) series
Colon and rectum	50 and over (women)	Every 1 year	Fecal immunochemical test
Liver	40 and over (high-risk group[a])	Every 6 months	Abdominal sonography and alpha fetoprotein (AFP)
Breast	40 and over (women)	Every 2 years	Mammography
Uterine cervix	20 and over (women)	Every 2 years	Conventional Pap smear test

Source: Suh et al. (2017)

[a]Those who are hepatitis B virus or hepatitis C virus carriers or have liver cirrhosis

Cancer Patients Management Program

To achieve standardization in palliative care, the Supporting and Evaluation Board of the Hospice-Palliative Care Program developed a national model of home-based and in-patient-based care in 2004. On the basis of these efforts, the Korean Government started supporting palliative care units in 2005 while simultaneously implementing the National Cancer Control Program for Terminal Cancer Care.

To provide systematic and appropriate medical care for the cancer patients in every community across the country, the Korean government has run a home-based cancer patient management program since 2001. The purpose of this program is to improve the quality of life for low-income cancer patients, thereby reducing the burden on their families. Public health centers are responsible for this initiative, while the NCC is in charge of planning, monitoring, and evaluating the program and offers training courses for healthcare providers (nurses, physicians, and other health professionals) (Choi, Han, Kim, Lim et al. 2017). The MOHW developed cancer pain control guidelines for healthcare providers and patients in 2004 and disseminates these guidelines on an annual basis.

The Financial Aid Program for Cancer Patients was designed to relieve the financial burden of cancer patients (Min, Yang, & Park, 2017). Starting with leukemia patients under 18 years in 2002, the program has expanded coverage to adult cancer patients within the following categories: (1) patients suffering from stomach, breast, cervical, liver, and colorectal cancers who participated in the NCSPs as a NHI beneficiary within the lower 50% income bracket; (2) lung cancer patients who are MAP recipients or NHI beneficiaries within the lower 50% income bracket; and (3) MAP beneficiaries.

In Korea, inequalities exist between Seoul and regional provinces in terms of cancer-related resources such as medical facilities and cancer specialists. Many cancer patients living in areas other than Seoul and its vicinity prefer visiting hospitals located in metropolitan cities including Seoul, which incurs additional expenses such as transportation and accommodation, which they must pay on their own. In order to eliminate this problem, in 2004, the government designated national university-affiliated hospitals in each province as regional cancer centers (RCCs). Nine RCCs were provided with financial support to strengthen their cancer care infrastructure and their eligibility for research grants, and, in 2011, three private university hospitals were added. The RCCs make significant contributions toward reducing cancer care inequalities in Korea and advancing regional cancer control activities.

Key Components of Leadership

Despite the relatively short period of time in which it was adopted, Korea's cancer control program has proven successful due to several factors. First, the government made a strong commitment to cancer prevention and control. Key stakeholders, such as government officials and politicians were willing to eliminate cancer. Through the development and revision, of the Cancer Control Act, strong legal support for the execution of all cancer control program was obtained, ensuring their stability and sustainability. In 2015, despite resistance from the public, they increased taxes on cigarettes to increase the national health promotion fund, which is the principal budget source of cancer control programs in Korea. Second, there is a well-established infrastructure for carrying out cancer control programs. The government established the NCC as a dedicated organization to oversee cancer control programs and established the KCCR, a nationwide cancer registration program essential for the prioritization, monitoring, and evaluation of program execution. This program is essential to evaluate the achievements of the various programs, ensuring that they are successfully meeting their mandates. Finally, it is necessary to consider how to combat this issue at the local and regional levels with Korean, instead of only at the national government level. Cancer control in each region is based on regional resources. Thus, efforts should be made to develop, network, and utilize local resources. In Korea, the NCC and RCC have been working together to train cancer-related experts and empower and motivate them to solve cancer issues at the local and regional levels. Furthermore, the Cancer Control Act of 2003, a legal framework for controlling cancer in Korea, promotes collaboration at the international level in order to be able to learn and share valuable lessons from other countries in terms of the latest evidence in cancer research and interventions, including participating in the International Agency for Cancer Research (IARC) since 2006 and establishing the National Cancer Center Graduate School of Cancer Science and Policy (NCC-GCSP) in 2014.

Future Directions

Despite successful cancer control consequences, there are still issues to be addressed. Efforts should be made to minimize program-related adverse effects and to improve their effectiveness and efficiency based on scientific evidence. In Korea, due to increasing participation of the NCSP, opportunistic screening has been implemented, and the problem of overdiagnosis and overtreatment of the thyroid cancer is emerging (Ahn, Kim, & Welch, 2014). In addition, more emphasis needs to be put on prevention. Addressing the leading risk factors for cancer, such as tobacco use, can help prevent cancers and other noncommunicable diseases. Additional resources should be allocated for programs that focus on prevention. Also, with the early diagnosis and development of treatment, the cancer survival rate is rapidly increasing. For example, the number of cancer survivors has recently exceeded one million (Jung et al., 2017). It is important to establish separate management policies for these. A Comprehensive Third-Term Cancer Control Plan (2016–2020) is being implemented to tackle these issues. This expands the extent of cancer patients from adults to children and adolescents and helps to develop and implement specific programs for cancer patients, as well as their caregivers and families.

References

Ahn, H. S., Kim, H. J., & Welch, H. G. (2014). Korea's thyroid-cancer "epidemic"–screening and over-diagnosis. *New England Journal of Medicine, 371*(19), 1765–1767.

Choi, J., Han, S., Kim, N., & Lim, Y. S. (2017). Increasing burden of liver cancer despite extensive use of antiviral agents in a hepatitis B virus-endemic population. *Hepatology, 66*(5), 1454–1463.

Choi, J. Y., Kong, K. A., Chang, Y. J., Jho, H. J., Ahn, E. M., Choi, S. K., et al. (2017). Effect of the duration of hospice and palliative care on the quality of dying and death in patients with terminal cancer: A nationwide multicenter study. *European Journal of Cancer Care, 27*(2), e12771. https://doi.org/10.1111/ecc.12771

CIA World Factbook. (2016). Retrieved March 22, 2018, from https://www.cia.gov/library/publications/the-world-factbook/.

Han, M. A., Choi, K. S., Park, J. H., Moor, M. A., & Park, E. C. (2011). Midcourse evaluation of the second-term 10-year plan for cancer control in Korea. *Asian Pacific Journal of Cancer Prevention, 12*(1), 327–333.

International Agency for Research on Cancer. (2017). *GLOBOCAN 2012*. Retrieved December 10, 2017, from http://globocan.iarc.fr/Default.aspx.

Jung, K. W., Won, Y. J., Oh, C. M., Kong, H. J., Lee, D. H., & Lee, K. H. (2017). Cancer statistics in Korea: Incidence, mortality, survival, and prevalence in 2014. *Cancer Research and Treatment, 49*(2), 292–305.

Kim, Y., Jun, J. K., Choi, K. S., Lee, H. Y., & Park, E. C. (2011). Overview of the National Cancer Screening Program and the cancer screening status in Korea. *Asian Pacific Journal of Cancer Prevention, 12*(3), 725–730.

Korea Centers for Disease Control & Prevention. (2017a). *Korea Health Statistics 2016*. Retrieved March 23, 2018, from http://knhanes.cdc.go.kr.

Korea Centers for Disease Control & Prevention. (2017b). *Korea Youth Risk Behavior Web-based Survey 2017*. Retrieved March 23, 2018, from http://yhs.cdc.go.kr.

Korea Centers for Disease Control & Prevention (2017c). *2015 National Health & Nutrition Survey*. Retrieved December 10, 2017, https://knhanes.cdc.go.kr/knhanes/sub03/sub03_01.do.

Korea Health Promotion Institute. (2017). *2014 HP2020 annual report*. Retrieved December 10, 2017, from http://www.khealth.or.kr/hp2020/bbsdtl.do?pgNo=&bbs_code=HB001&bbs_ix=13&pageIndex=1.

Korean Statistical Information Service. (2017). *Deaths and Death rates by cause*. Retrieved December 10, 2017, from http://kosis.kr/eng/search/search01_List.jsp.

Kye, S. Y., Lee, M. H., Yoo, J., Oh, K., & Jun, J. K. (2017). Factors affecting the satisfaction of cancer information of the social network services in Korea. *Epidemiology and Health, 39*, e2017057. https://doi.org/10.4178/epih.e2017057

Kye, S. Y., Park, E. Y., Oh, K., & Park, K. (2015). Perceptions of cancer risk and cause of cancer risk in Korean adults. *Cancer Research and Treatment, 47*(2), 158–165.

Kye, S. Y., Yoo, J., Lee, M. H., & Jun, J. K. (2015). Effects of a cancer prevention advertisement on beliefs and knowledge about cancer prevention. *Asian Pacific Journal of Cancer Prevention, 16*(14), 5793–5800.

Lee, W. C., Shin, H. R., & Kim, C. M. (2001). Establishing cancer screening recommendations for major cancers in Korea. *Journal of Korean Medical Association, 45*(8), 959–963 in Korean.

Ma, D., Sakai, H., Wakabayashi, C., Kwon, J. S., Lee, Y., Liu, S., et al. (2017). The prevalence and risk factor control associated with non-communicable diseases in China, Japan, and Korea. *Journal of Epidemiology, 27*(12), 568–573.

Min, H. S., Yang, H., & Park, K. (2017). Supporting low-income cancer patients: Recommendations for the Public Financial Aid Program in the Republic of Korea. *Cancer Research and Treatment*. https://doi.org/10.4143/crt.2017.401

National Cancer Center. (2017). *About NCC*. Retrieved December 10, 2017, from http://ncc.re.kr/main.ncc?uri=english/sub01_Greetings.

Oh, J. K., Lim, M. K., Yun, E. H., Shin, S. H., Park, E. Y., & Park, E. C. (2013). Cost and effectiveness of the nationwide government-supported smoking cessation clinics in the Republic of Korea. *Tobacco Control, 22*(e1), e73–e77.

Park, B., Jung, K. W., Oh, C. M., Choi, K. S., Suh, M., & Jun, J. K. (2015). Ten-year changes in the hepatitis B prevalence in the birth cohorts in Korea: Results from nationally representative cross-sectional surveys. *Medicine, 94*(41), e1469.

Suh, M., Song, S., Cho, H. N., Park, B., Jun, J. K., Choi, E., et al. (2017). Trends in participation rates for the National Cancer Screening Program in Korea, 2002-2012. *Cancer Research and Treatment, 49*(3), 798–806.

United Nations. (2016). *Human development report*. Retrieved March 22, 2018, from http://hdr.undp.org/sites/default/files/2016_human_development_report.pdf.

WHO Statistical Profile. (2015). Retrieved March 22, 2018, from http://www.who.int/countries/en/

Yoo, K. Y. (2007). Cancer Control Activities in the Republic of Korea. *Japanese Journal of Clinical Oncology, 38*(5), 327–333.

Yun, E. H., Lim, M. K., Oh, J. K., Ki, I. H., Shin, S. H., & Jeong, B. Y. (2016). Quitline activity in the Republic of Korea. *Asian Pacific Journal of Cancer Prevention, 17*(S2), 1–5.

Discussion Questions

1. What are the major strengths of Korea's national cancer control program? What about weaknesses or deficiencies?
2. What challenges may inhibit progress in cancer control in Korea or globally in the next two decades?
3. Are there similarities in cancer prevention and control strategies across countries? Why do specific cultural contexts require tailoring of programs addressing cancer across countries?
4. What priority actions are needed for your own country to reduce its burden of cancer?
5. Who are the major stakeholders in cancer-related programs? Can the international community get more involved in cancer prevention and control at the global level? How might this be done?

Follow-Up Reading

Jun, J. K., Choi, K. S., Lee, H. Y., Suh, M., Park, B., Song, S. H., et al. (2017). Effectiveness of the Korean National Cancer Screening Program in reducing gastric cancer mortality. *Gastroenterology, 152*(6), 1319–1328.

Park, S., Oh, C. M., Cho, H., Lee, J. Y., Jung, K. W., Jun, J. K., et al. (2016). Association between screening and the thyroid cancer "epidemic" in South Korea: Evidence from a nationwide study. *British Medical Journal, 355*, i5745.

Runowicz, C. D., Leach. C., Henry, N. L., Henry, K. S., Mackey, H. T., Cowens-Alvarado, R. L., et al. (2015). American Cancer Society/American Society of Clinical Oncology breast cancer survivorship care guideline. *CA: A Cancer Journal for Clinicians, 66*(1), 43–73. National Cancer Institute.

National Cancer Moonshot Initiative. National Cancer Institute. Available from https://www.cancer.gov/research/key-initiatives/moonshot-cancer-initiative.

Chapter 12
Protecting Filipino Overseas Migrant Workers

Jorge V. Tigno

Philippines: Demographics overview
Population: 104,256,076
Life expectancy: 69.2 years

- Male: 65.7
- Female: 72.9

GNI per capita: $8395
Total fertility rate: 3.02 children/woman
Under-five mortality rate (per 1000 live births): 30
UN HDI: 0.682
Top 3 causes of death:

- Ischemic heart disease
- Stroke
- Lower respiratory infections

Source: CIA World Factbook (2016), UNDP Human Development Programme (2016), WHO publications (2015)

This chapter provides a description of the overseas Filipino workforce, an overview of the programs in place through five national agencies for overseas nationals, and an analysis of the factors that led to the Philippine government developing a comprehensive protection program for its workers abroad. The combined programs, delivered via government agencies to assist with the strategic

J. V. Tigno (✉)
Department of Political Science, University of the Philippines–Diliman,
Quezon City, Philippines
e-mail: jorge.tigno@upd.edu.ph

© Springer Nature Switzerland AG 2019
M. Withers, J. McCool (eds.), *Global Health Leadership*,
https://doi.org/10.1007/978-3-319-95633-6_12

management of labor migration, have become a hallmark of the Philippine model. Finally, this chapter will present a brief analysis of possible future steps that the Philippine government could take to mitigate the social costs of migration.

Introduction

The Philippines is known worldwide for its skilled, highly mobile, adaptable workforce. The country ranks high in human capital terms compared to many of its neighboring countries in Southeast Asia (Philippine Star, 2017). Many Filipino migrant workers leave their country after having achieved high levels of education and professional training (Sayres, 2007). Over the past four decades, the Philippine government (in particular, the Department of Labor) has played a significant role in efforts to manage labor mobility while promoting the country as a leading exporter of labor worldwide (Martin, Abella, & Midgley, 2004). For the last decade, the country has deployed approximately one million migrant workers every year (see Fig. 12.1). Overseas migrant workers are those who plan to eventually return to their countries, as opposed to permanent migrants who move permanently to another country. Estimate of Filipino migrant workers living and working abroad is approximately ten million, or about 10% of the total population (Asis, 2017). Yet the level of expertise distributed across the migrant workforce is confined to low-skilled work categories, such as manual laborers and domestic helpers.

Filipino migrant workers are employed in over a hundred countries worldwide but mostly confined to specific countries in the Middle East (e.g., Saudi Arabia,

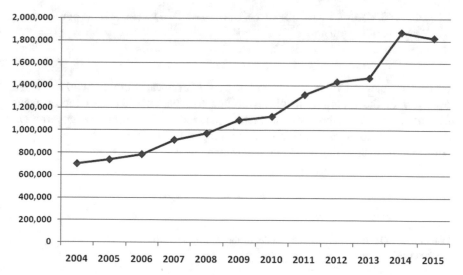

Fig. 12.1 Annual deployment of land-based Filipino migrant workers. Source: (POEA, 2015)

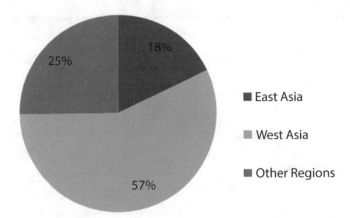

Fig. 12.2 Percentage distribution of Filipino migrant worker by region. Source: (Philippine Statistics Authority, 2016)

Qatar, Kuwait, and the United Arab Emirates) and East Asia (e.g., Hong Kong, Taiwan, Japan, Singapore, and South Korea) (Fig. 12.2).

Frequent natural disasters, economic and political instability, rapid population growth and urbanization, and low salaries are the push factors most commonly cited for why people leave the Philippines to work abroad (Battistella, 1992; Asis, 2017). Overseas migration is also a tradition, with roots in the Spanish colonization of the Philippines and the Spanish-American war following which the Philippines became a territory of the USA. The first generation of Filipino workers moved to Hawaii in 1906 to work on fruit plantations; this trend has continued ever since (Asis, 2017). Many Filipinos now seek employment abroad as a means to earn enough income to support their families who remain in the Philippines in an effort to lift them out of poverty (Ducanes & Abella, 2008).

The consequences of labor migration among the working-age population are significant for the Philippines. As a result of massive deployments, the country has become a major receiver of income remittances from overseas migrants. The annual income derived from remittances has been steadily increasing since the early 2000s (Fig. 12.3). The Philippines now ranks third after India and China as major global recipients of remittances (Asis, 2017). In 2016, the country received nearly US$27 billion in remittance earnings, considerably higher than the amount of overseas development assistance (ODA) and foreign direct investments (FDIs) combined (BSP, 2016).

Given their higher educational attainment and income potential as compared to the Philippine-based workforce, Filipino overseas migrant workers may be perceived as relatively privileged and better prepared to address the many uncertainties of everyday life in other countries (Ducanes & Abella, 2008). However, migrant workers also face numerous challenges and are particularly vulnerable to exploitation (Center for Migrant Advocacy, 2016; Torres, 2017; Tan, 2018). The "OFWs" (or "overseas Filipino workers," as they are popularly called) have to endure challenges ranging from loneliness and isolation to racial and sexual

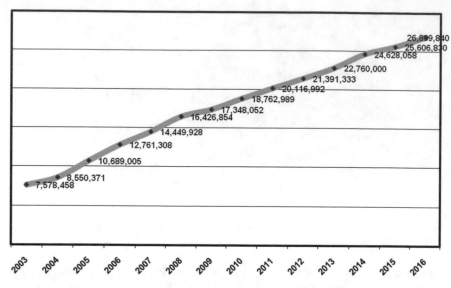

26,899,840
25,606,830
24,628,058
22,760,000
21,391,333
20,116,992
18,762,989
17,348,052
16,426,854
14,449,928
12,761,308
10,689,005
8,550,371
7,578,458

2003 2004 2005 2006 2007 2008 2009 2010 2011 2012 2013 2014 2015 2016

Fig. 12.3 Annual remittances of Filipino migrant workers (US$). Source: (BSP, 2016)

discrimination and even physical and mental abuse. In addition, many also face work-related problems such as nonpayment of their salaries by exploitative brokers and employers, long working hours, and unhealthy work environments. The growth of private labor recruitment agencies has exacerbated these problems (Asis, 2017). This precarious situation is compounded by the predominance of employment being performed in the so-called "3D" (dirty, dangerous, and difficult) and low-skilled occupations, such as domestic helpers, factory workers, caregivers, and entertainers. These roles are characterized by low pay and minimal bargaining power for employees. Migrant workers' vulnerabilities are further compounded when employed in countries afflicted by armed conflict, natural disaster, and/or disease outbreaks (IOM, 2012).

In response to the unique challenges faced by migrant workers, the Philippine government has attempted to provide systematic, timely, and effective initiatives to protect migrant workers' welfare abroad (Chavez & Piper, 2015). The Philippine government has recognized the benefits of outbound labor migration and has attempted to limit the risks by establishing various mechanisms of support. Over the last four decades, the government has established institutions dedicated to serving the welfare needs of migrant workers and their families in the Philippines (Orbeta, Abrigo, & Cabalfin, 2009). Since 1974, public institutions like the Philippine Overseas Employment Administration (POEA) and the Overseas Workers Welfare Administration (OWWA) have overseen the systematic and large-scale deployment of migrant workers for overseas jobs. These efforts have proven to be an effective starting point for change.

Program Description

The Legal and Operational Framework for Protecting Filipino Migrant Workers

Philippine Labor Migration Policy historically focused on removing barriers for migrant workers to increase accessibility of employment abroad by facilitating recruitment and necessary paperwork to support Filipinos who want to work abroad but were not necessarily focused on the protection of their rights. The origins of the overseas employment program (as labor migration has come to be known in the Philippines) can be traced back to 1974 with the promulgation of the New Labor Code. Presidential Decree 442 (otherwise known as the 1974 Labor Code) formalized the overseas employment program. No previous government program addressing labor migration came close to matching the comprehensive nature of the 1974 Labor Code; previous enactments were piecemeal and short-sighted. In particular, the Code institutionalized labor migration through legislation and established a more proactive and strategic government effort.

At the same time, technical advisors and experts in the Department of Labor and Employment (DOLE) began to appreciate the potential of labor export in reducing the high unemployment rates and contributing to the achievement of full employment rates for the Philippines. Early studies were conducted to monitor overseas employment patterns and their development contributions. For instance, Abella (1976) observed that the remittances sent by Filipinos working overseas in 1974 were higher than the Philippines' combined earnings for that year from its two major export crops at the time—sugar and copra (Menjivar, DaVanzo, Greenwell, & Valdez, 1998).

The purpose of the 1974 Labor Code was to develop an overseas employment program that would ensure the efficient and effective utilization and market potential of the country's surplus human resource, without jeopardizing the security and best possible working and living conditions for migrant workers. Since 1974, other policies have emerged that reflect the urgent need to better manage labor outflows. In 1995, the Overseas Filipinos and Migrant Workers Act (Republic Actor RA 8042, 1995) was enacted to "institute the policies of overseas employment and establish a higher standard of protection and promotion of the welfare of migrant workers and their families and overseas Filipinos in distress." Some of the services that the law mandates include:

- Issuance of travel advisories and information on labor and employment conditions and migration to be published three times a quarter, in general circulation newspapers, to prevent illegal recruitment practices
- Emergency Repatriation Fund for repatriation of migrant workers in times of crisis, such as war, epidemic, or disasters
- Establishment of Migrant Workers and Other Overseas Filipinos Resource Center which provides legal services, medical services, post-arrival orientation,

settlement and community networking services, human resource development, and daily monitoring of migrant workers' situations
- Establishment of a replacement and monitoring center to support the reintegration of returning Filipino migrant workers into Philippine society through livelihood programs and promoting local employment, among other services
- Legal Assistance Fund to provide legal services to Filipino migrant workers and overseas Filipinos in distress

The Philippines labor migration management system has also differentiated the institutional mechanisms of care and assistance provided to migrant workers. For example, the Philippine Overseas Employment Administration (POEA) is primarily tasked with licensing private recruitment entities and regulating their operations. It is also responsible for certifying the labor contracts of migrant workers, which requires them to ensure they are operating at an acceptable standard. The Overseas Workers Welfare Administration (OWWA) is tasked with providing welfare related-services to migrant workers in crisis and in vulnerable situations through the Philippine embassy or international consulate. Both the POEA and OWWA are embedded within the Philippine Department of Labor and Employment (DOLE). The DOLE is also given the task of setting up Philippine Overseas Labor Offices in areas where there are concentrations of Filipino migrant workers, which are headed by the labor attaché for that country. There are currently about 36 Philippine Overseas Labor Offices worldwide (DOLE, 2016). The Department of Foreign Affairs (DFA) is also mandated by law to provide on-site services and interventions through its embassies and consulates.

In addition to the Department of Labor and the Department of Foreign Affairs, various other government agencies are also tasked to provide support to Filipino nationals while abroad. These include the Department of Social Welfare and Development (for situations involving women and minors), the Bureau of Immigration (which helps facilitates the repatriation and return of migrant workers), and the Department of Health (which monitors any potential health risks). Another unique feature of the Philippine government response to labor-related challenges encountered by migrant workers overseas is the establishment of Migrant Resource Centers in countries with expatriate Filipino communities (Section 19 of RA 8042). These Resource Centers are mandated to offer counseling and legal services, assistance for those seeking medical and hospital care, information on return and resettlement back to the Philippines, and other services that can mitigate labor and welfare issues. In addition, pre-departure seminars are offered by private recruitment agencies, the government, and civil society groups and are designed to help migrant workers prepare for the challenges of being overseas, such as providing rudimentary language training as well as information on cultural differences (Tigno, 2013). These agencies also enable the linkage between migrant workers and government agencies in times of emergency where response protocols in crises are required.

Key Components of Leadership

In a 2017 report, the World Bank stated "The highly-developed support system for migrant labor in the Philippines can serve as a model for other countries" (World Bank, 2017). The success of this model can be attributed to several factors, including the fact that the migrant protection system is now more rights-based (Chavez & Piper, 2015). In general, government agencies have followed an operational framework based on providing humanitarian assistance to migrant workers and on the concept of employee empowerment. Extra emphasis has also been placed on adherence to established international labor conventions and standards like the Forced Labor Convention (1930), the Freedom of Association and Protection of the Right to Organize Convention (1948), the Equal Remuneration Convention (1951), and the Discrimination Convention (1958), among others. In addition, Philippine labor migration policies provide that Filipino migrant workers can only work in countries that afford adequate protective guarantees for the rights of all their workers (local and foreign) or are "taking positive, concrete measures to protect the rights of migrant workers." In 2011, the government issued a ban on sending workers to 41 countries because the countries concerned had failed to sign agreements to protect foreign workers from abuse (MacGeown, 2011). Most recently, in 2018, the Philippine government offered free flights home to the 10,000 Filipinos who had overstayed their visa in Kuwait after the body of their compatriot 29-year-old Joanna Demafelis was found in the freezer of her employers' home (BBC, 2018). A ban on the deployment of overseas foreign workers to Kuwait followed after the deaths of Demafelis and several other women (Berlinger & Jorgio, 2018; Rey, 2018).

In addition, the Philippine government has endeavored to make the protection and promotion of the rights and welfare of Filipino migrant workers a priority. Several factors explain the rationale behind this emphasis. First, the country has become heavily dependent on the remittance earnings of its OFW workforce. The revenue generated through annual remittances received by the Philippines government greatly outweighs both the foreign investment and development assistance. Extending government assistance to overseas nationals can be interpreted as a strategic way for the Philippines to protect the economic benefits of an international workforce. Benefits realized in the real estate and retail trade sectors, for example, are a tangible by-product of income received by migrant workers' families through remittances, as this affords extra disposable income to purchase properties and merchandise that nonmigrant families may not be able to afford (Reyes, 2017; Ducanes, 2015).

Second, the impetus to provide formal protection to migrant workers abroad was a long process punctuated by events like the case of Flor Contemplacion. In 1995, Contemplacion, a Filipino maid in Singapore, was charged and convicted of murdering her young ward and was later hanged. Many Filipinos thought she was innocent of the charges which prompted outrage against Singapore and several Philippine officials (Vines, 1995; Shenon, 1995). Many Filipinos also thought the Philippine government should have done more to protect her rights as a migrant.

High-profile events like the Contemplacion case placed legislators under pressure to institute measures to protect migrant workers (Schmetzer, 1995).

Third, the sociopolitical situation in the Philippines post-1986 which restored democracy to the country saw civil society groups become openly critical of government ineptitude and inefficiencies (Clarke, 2013). Repressed, yet outraged by many years of authoritarian rule, the free media now made it possible to raise the awareness of government inaction (Coronel, 2001). Transparency and accountability in government became paramount, at least among citizens.

Challenges

In many ways, the Philippine overseas employment program has been described as a global model in labor migration management (Orbeta Jr & Abrigo, 2011). Leadership demonstrated by Philippines government and allied agencies, both public and private, have shaped the Filipino labor outbound migration phenomenon. Migration was openly acknowledged as being critical to the country's economic development. In the past decade, migration governance in the Philippines has gone beyond labor migration policies and remittances, instead working toward linking migration policies to broader development goals. In 2014, the National Economic and Development Authority (NEDA), the government's key planning agency, established a Subcommittee on Migration and Development to improve coordination among government agencies and devote more attention to migration and development. The last two national Philippine Development Plans have incorporated migration into national development planning. Migration Resource Centers and similar structures in local government units have been established in selected regional and local governments (Asis, 2017).

Despite this progress, several challenges remain. First, specifically, there is a need for existing government agencies to be more sensitive to the long-term development implications of overseas employment. Migration should be a safe, viable choice for people, one of many options to improve living standards, and not an imperative, or the only viable option for development. Philippine President Benigno Aquino III (2010–2016) was especially outspoken about the importance of migration; his social contract with the Filipino people is expressed in the following statement:

"from a government that treats its people as an export commodity and as a means to foreign exchange, disregarding the social cost to Filipino families, to a government that creates jobs at home, so that working abroad will be a choice rather than a necessity; and when its citizens do choose to become OFWs, their welfare and protection will still be the government's priority." (Asis, 2017)

The 2017–2022 Philippine Development Plan acknowledges that "limited employment opportunities force Filipinos to migrate by necessity and not by choice." Unemployment and underemployment remain challenges, and the report highlights the need to address underemployment, youth unemployment, low labor market participation of women, and inadequate jobs leading to out-migration (National Economic and Development Authority, 2017). A review of the country's educational system could help ensure that the appropriate combination of skills and competencies is being achieved to meet the changing demands of internal and external labor markets in the future.

Second, although remittances offer benefits for the country, over the long-term, there are risks associated with this process. Many have been critical of the reliance on remittances, believing that the large amounts of remittances have facilitated the drain of educated workers abroad and have inhibited motivation to improve conditions within the country. For example, out-migration of Filipino nurses has created a shortage of nurses locally (ILO, 2015). Others believe that reliance on remittances may have delayed the implementation of needed reforms (Asis, 2017).

Future Directions

More efforts are needed to protect workers' rights abroad. Working conditions abroad vary depending on whether the host country acknowledges and enforces international labor standards outlined by the International Labor Organization (ILO), a United Nations agency (ILO, 2010). However, although the ILO can register complaints, it does not have the authority to impose penalties or sanctions on governments that do not comply. Measures to protect worker's rights should also ensure that the employment institutions support Filipino workers to achieve appropriate level employment in their host country reflective of their skills and experience (Orbeta Jr & Abrigo, 2011; Pernia, 2011).

Continued focus on improving services for the reintegration of those returning from overseas, many of whom have been abroad for years, remains paramount (World Bank, 2017). Many Filipino migrant workers return with no concrete plans for employment or savings; they often struggle to find work at home. Some return to strained family relationships resulting from estrangement; some return disillusioned from their experiences abroad or from not meeting personal financial or career goals. Returning OFWs often experience emotional distress from difficulties readjusting to life at home or from broken ties with their families and communities (ILO, 2015). In addition, families that relied upon regular remittances from the family member abroad now have to adapt to the loss of that income (ILO, 2015).

Conclusion

The Philippines is one of the top global exporters of labor. Migration can have many positive consequences to both the sending and receiving countries. Yet, migrant workers are often vulnerable to exploitation and abuse while abroad. Historically, the Philippine Labor Migration Policy focused on removing barriers for overseas workers to increase accessibility for employment abroad. However, over the past four decades, the Philippine government has instituted a comprehensive set of laws and services available to overseas workers before, during, and after they migrate. The Philippine labor migration management system has, arguably, had a profound impact on shaping the Filipino labor out-migration phenomenon. Although there are areas for improvement, historical developments in labor migration policy enacted by the Philippine government demonstrate the wide-reaching impact of government-led leadership protecting the rights of migrant workers. Further analysis and policy responses are also required to address the factors that drive outbound migration and the consequences of this phenomenon.

References

Abella, M. (1976). Export of Filipino manpower: A question of competitive advantage. *Philippine Labor Review, 1*(2), 89–94.

Asis, M.M.B. (2017). *Beyond labor migration toward development and (possibly) return.* Retrieved February 25, 2018, from https://www.migrationpolicy.org/article/philippines-beyond-labor-migration-toward-development-and-possibly-return.

Bangko Sentral ng Pilipinas (BSP). (2016). *Statistics.* Retrieved December 20, 2017, from http://www.bsp.gov.ph/statistics/efs_ext3.asp.

Battistella, G. (1992). *Philippine labor migration: impact and policy.* Quezon City: Scalabrini Migration Center.

BBC News. (2018). *Joanna Demafelis: Employers of Filipina maid found dead in freezer arrested.* Retrieved March 18, 2018, from http://www.bbc.com/news/world-middle-east-43177349.

Berlinger, J., & Jorgio, J. (2018). *Killing prompts return of Philippines workers from Kuwait.* Retrieved February 24, 2018, from https://www.cnn.com/2018/02/13/asia/philippines-domestic-workers-intl/index.html.

Center for Migrant Advocacy. (2016). *Protection of OFWs, especially domestic workers, urgently needed.* Retrieved February 12, 2018, from http://globalnation.inquirer.net/141983/protection-of-ofws-especially-domestic-workers-urgently-needed#ixzz56sgtsnHr.

Central Intelligence Agency (CIA). (2016). *CIA World Factbook.* Retrieved February April 11, 2018, from https://www.cia.gov/library/publications/the-world-factbook/

Chavez, J. J., & Piper, N. (2015). The reluctant leader: The Philippine journey from labor export to championing a rights-based approach to overseas employment. In E. Berman & S. Haque (Eds.), *Asian leadership in policy and governance (public policy and governance, Volume 24)* (pp. 305–344). Wagon Lane, Bingley: Emerald Group Publishing Limited.

Clarke, G. (2013). *Civil society in the Philippines; theoretical, methodological, and policy debates.* Abingdon and New York: Routledge.

Coronel, S. (2001). The media, the market, and democracy: The case of the Philippines. *The Public, 8*(2), 109–126.

Department of Labor and Employment (DOLE). (2016). *Directory—Philippine overseas labor offices.* Retrieved January 3, 2018, from https://www.dole.gov.ph/pages/view/24.

Ducanes, G. (2015). The welfare impact of overseas migration on Philippine households: Analysis using panel data. *Asian and Pacific Migration Journal, 24*(1), 79–106.

Ducanes, G., & Abella, M. (2008). *Overseas Filipino workers and their impact on household poverty.* International Labour Organization (ILO) Working paper no.8. International Labour Office; ILO Regional Office for Asia and the Pacific, Asian Regional Programme on Governance of Labour Migration, Bangkok.

International Labour Organization (ILO). (2010). *International labour migration: A rights based approach.* Retrieved April 11, 2018, from http://www.ilo.org/wcmsp5/groups/public/%2D%2D-ed_protect/%2D%2D-protrav/%2D%2D-migrant/documents/publication/wcms_208594.pdf.

International Labour Organization (ILO). (2015). *Return and reintegration to the Philippines: An information guide for migrant Filipino health workers.* Retrieved February 24, 2018, from http://www.ilo.org/wcmsp5/groups/public/%2D%2D-asia/%2D%2D-ro-bangkok/%2D%2D-ilo-manila/documents/publication/wcms_367738.pdf.

International Organisation for Migration (IOM). (2012). *IOM migration crisis operational framework.* Retrieved December 20, 2017, from https://www.iom.int/files/live/sites/iom/files/What-We-Do/docs/MC2355_-_IOM_Migration_Crisis_Operational_Framework.pdf.

MacGeown, K. (2011). Philippines bans its workers from 41 countries. *BBC News.* Retrieved February 12, 2018, from http://www.bbc.com/news/world-asia-15561596.

Martin, P., Abella, M., & Midgley, E. (2004). Best practices to manage migration: The Philippines. *The International Migration Review, 38*(4), 1544–1560.

Menjivar, C., DaVanzo, J., Greenwell, L., & Valdez, R. B. (1998). Remittance Behavior among Salvadoran and Filipino Immigrants in Los Angeles. *The International Migration Review, 32*(1), 97–126.

National Economic and Development Authority. (2017). *Philippines development plan 2017-2022.* Retrieved February 25, 2018, from http://pdp.neda.gov.ph/wp-content/uploads/2017/01/PDP-2017-2022-07-20-2017.pdf.

Orbeta, A. Jr. & Abrigo, M. (2011). *Managing international labor migration: The Philippine experience.* Philippine Institute for Development Studies (PIDS) Discussion Paper Series 2011-33. Retrieved December 4, 2017, from https://dirp4.pids.gov.ph/webportal/CDN/PUBLICATIONS/pidspjd11-philippines.pdf.

Orbeta, A. Jr., Abrigo, M., Cabalfin, M. (2009). *Institutions serving Philippine international labor migrants.* Philippine Institute for Development Studies Discussion Paper Series no. 2009-31. Retrieved December 22, 2017, from https://dirp3.pids.gov.ph/ris/dps/pidsdps0931.pdf.

Pernia, E. (2011). Is labour export good development policy? *The Philippine Review of Economics, 48*(1), 13–34.

Philippine Overseas Employment Administration (POEA) (2015). *OFW Statistics.* Retrieved December 22, 2017, from http://www.poea.gov.ph/ofwstat/ofwstat.html.

Philippine Star. (2017). In charts: How the Philippines fares in Southeast Asia. *Philippine Star.* Retrieved February 12, 2018, from https://beta.philstar.com/headlines/2017/11/11/1757872/charts-how-philippines-fares-southeast-asia#k8orDo7KWWXIYbpd.99.

Philippine Statistics Authority (PSA). (2016). *Survey of Overseas Filipinos 2016.* Retrieved December 21, 2017, from https://psa.gov.ph/content/statistical-tables-overseas-filipino-workers-ofw-2016.

Republic Act 8042. (1995). *Migrant workers and overseas Filipinos Act of 1995.* Manila.

Rey, A. (2018). Philippines bans workers' deployment to Kuwait. *Rappler.* Retrieved February 12, 2018, from https://www.rappler.com/nation/195827-philippines-total-deployment-ban-ofws-kuwait.

Reyes, R.R. (2017). Property sector to sustain growth momentum in 2017. *Business Mirror.* Retrieved January 3, 2018, from https://businessmirror.com.ph/property-sector-sustain-growth-momentum-2017/.

Sayres, N.J. (2007). *An analysis of the situation of Filipino domestic workers.* Geneva: International Labor Organization. Retrieved February 12, 2018, from http://www.ilo.org/wcmsp5/groups/public/@asia/@ro-bangkok/@ilo-manila/documents/publication/wcms_124895.pdf.

Schmetzer, U. (1995). Anger at maid's death abroad now Shakes Filipino Oligarchy. *Chicago Tribune.* Retrieved February 12, 2018, from http://articles.chicagotribune.com/1995-04-06/news/9504060181_1_flor-contemplacion-filipino-saudi-arabia.

Shenon, P. (1995). Filipinos protest Singapore death sentence. *The New York Times.* Retrieved February 12, 2018, from http://www.nytimes.com/1995/03/16/world/filipinos-protest-singapore-death-sentence.html.

Tan, L. (2018). Jail, home detention for Filipino restaurateurs over exploitation of workers in Auckland. *New Zealand Herald.* Retrieved February 12, 2018, from http://www.nzherald.co.nz/nz/news/article.cfm?c_id=1&objectid=11990563.

Tigno, J. (2013). Gendered protection and care: Pre-departure orientation for migrant women from the Philippines. In J. Tigno (Ed.), *Interrogating migration: New questions and emerging trends in the Philippines* (pp. 151–182). Quezon City: Philippine Migration Research Network and Philippine Social Science Council.

Torres, E. (2017). What will it take to protect Filipino domestic workers from abuse and exploitation in the Middle East?. *Equal Times.* Retrieved February 12, 2018, from https://www.equal-times.org/what-will-it-take-to-protect?lang=en#.WoFIsK6Wbcs.

United Nations Development Programme (UNDP). (2016). *Human development report.* Retrieved April 11, 2018, from http://hdr.undp.org/sites/default/files/2016_human_development_report.pdf.

Vines, S. (1995). Philippines set for `innocent' verdict on hanged maid. *Independent.* Retrieved February 12, 2018, from http://www.independent.co.uk/news/world/philippines-set-for-innocent-verdict-on-hanged-maid-1613888.html.

World Bank. (2017). *Migrating to opportunity: Overcoming barriers to labor mobility in Southeast Asia.* Retrieved February 23, 2018, from http://www.worldbank.org/en/region/eap/publication/migrating-to-opportunity-overcoming-barriers-to-labor-mobility-in-southeast-asia.

World Health Organisation (WHO). (2015). Retrieved April 11, 2018, from http://www.who.int/countries/en/.

Discussion Questions

1. Migration has negative connotations but migrants also contribute positively to both the sending and receiving countries. Name at least three of the benefits of migration.
2. Why do people move? List the three major reasons for why people would want to leave and settle in another country. How do the motivations to migrate differ among groups?
3. What are the historical roots of outbound migration in the Philippines? What strategies could the Philippine government employ to improve the local conditions that contribute to the desire to work abroad? And what are the reasons why the government might not implement these strategies?
4. Name five challenges that migrant workers might face when settling in their country of destination. How can the government prevent or reduce the problems that migrant workers face? Suggest at least two interventions that the receiving country's government could implement that would provide enhanced support for migrant workers.
5. What would effective, ethical labor migration look like at the regional level? What are the likely challenges that intergovernmental institutions like the Association of Southeast Asian Nations (ASEAN) and the European Union (EU) need to overcome in order to achieve this?

Follow-Up Reading

Orbeta, A. Jr., Abrigo, M., & Cabalfin, M. (2009). *Institutions Serving Philippine International Labor Migrants.* Philippine Institute for Development Studies Discussion Paper Series No. 2009–31. Available from https://dirp3.pids.gov.ph/ris/dps/pidsdps0931.pdf.

Asis, M. M. B., & Baggio, F. (Eds.). (2008). *Moving out, back and up: International Migration and Development Prospects in the Philippines.* Quezon City: Scalabrini Migration Center.

Ducanes, G. (2015). The welfare impact of overseas migration on Philippine households: Analysis using panel data. *Asian and Pacific Migration Journal 24*(1), 79–106.

Encinas-Franco, J. (2015). Overseas Filipino Workers (OFWs) as Heroes: Discursive Origins of the "Bagong Bayani" in the Era of Labor Export. *Humanities Diliman 12*(2), 56–78.

International Organization for Migration (IOM) and Scalabrini Migration Center (SMC) (2013). *Country Migration Report*, The Philippines 2013. Makati City: IOM.

Orbeta, A. Jr., &Abrigo, M. R. (2011). *Managing International Labor Migration: The Philippine Experience*. Philippine Institute for Development Studies (PIDS) Discussion Paper Series 2011–33. Available from https://dirp4.pids.gov.ph/webportal/CDN/PUBLICATIONS/pidspjd11-philippines.pdf.

Zosa, V., & Orbeta, A. Jr. (2009). *The Social and Economic Impact of Philippine International Labor*.

Migration and Remittances. Philippine Institute for Development Studies (PIDS) Discussion Paper Series no 0.2009–32. Available from https://dirp4.pids.gov.ph/ris/dps/pidsdps0932.pdf.

Chapter 13
mHealth in the Pacific Rim: Leadership Through Technology-Based Interventions

Judith McCool, Rosie Dobson, Elaine Umali, Linda Cameron, and Robyn Whittaker

Samoa: Demographics Overview
Population: 200,108
Life expectancy: 74 years

- Male: 71.1
- Female: 77

GNI per capita: $5372
Total fertility rate: 4.1 children/woman
Under-five mortality rate (per 1000 live births): 17.5
UN HDI: 0.704
Top 3 causes of death:

- Cardiovascular diseases
- Respiratory diseases
- Diabetes mellitus

Source: CIA World Factbook (2016), UNDP Human Development Programme (2016), WHO publications (2015)

J. McCool (✉)
School of Population Health, University of Auckland, Auckland, New Zealand
e-mail: j.mccool@auckland.ac.nz

R. Dobson · R. Whittaker
National Institute for Health Innovation, University of Auckland, Auckland, New Zealand

E. Umali
University of Auckland, Auckland, New Zealand

L. Cameron
Department of Psychology, University of California, Merced, CA, USA

© Springer Nature Switzerland AG 2019
M. Withers, J. McCool (eds.), *Global Health Leadership*,
https://doi.org/10.1007/978-3-319-95633-6_13

About three-quarters of the world's population have access to a mobile phone. In the last decade alone, the number of mobile subscriptions have grown from fewer than one billion to over six billion, of which nearly five billion are from low- and middle-income countries (LMICs) (World Bank, 2018). The increased access to mobile phones and network coverage has introduced the opportunity to innovate how we deliver health services. Mobile phones offer advantages for communities who are remote, disengaged, or hard-to-reach, for various reasons. In an era of Universal Health Coverage, as a goal within the UN Sustainable Development Goals (SDG), leadership in healthcare delivery is essential. To achieve the ambitious SDG targets set at the global level, business as usual is no longer feasible. New modes of communication are now, more than ever, indispensable to enabling equitable access to health services, including health promoting message support.

Mobile health (hereafter mHealth) is defined provisionally by the World Health Organization as a "medical and public health practice supported by mobile devices"; it "involves the use and capitalisation on a mobile phone's core utility of voice and short messaging service (SMS) as well as more complex functionalities" (WHO, 2011). One of the formative trials of mHealth for tobacco cessation support provided evidence of the potential value of a simple text message to affect behavior change. In this work, Rogers et al. (2005) identified that smokers who received text message support, developed in accordance with the theory of behavior change, were twice as likely to quit smoking. This early trial of text message support for tobacco cessation was groundbreaking. Since then, developments in the application of mHealth, including text message and smartphone applications (apps) to improve disease surveillance and service delivery to behavior change, have burgeoned.

mHealth has evolved from its origins in clinical medicine to a broader application aimed at improving innovation and access to information for population health. The use of mHealth in LMICs has increased substantially over the past 5 years, driven partially by increased access to mobile networks and affordable handsets (Umali, McCool, & Whittaker, 2016). In low-resourced settings, mobile telecommunication services are among the most prominently advertised consumer products. Mobile technology for development purposes has also become a core focus for international telecommunications governance networks, driven in part by the potential for accessing new, previously underserved populations (International Telecommunications Union, 2017). Despite the inherent challenges associated with public–private partnerships in health, they are essential for mHealth. The reliance on the telecommunications providers (or intermediaries called gateway providers who route messages between the sender and receiver) is essential to delivering targeted, scalable, cost-effective mobile phone-based interventions. There is significant potential for mobile phones to support the delivery of some core components of Universal Health Coverage, which is fundamental to the achievement of the SDGs. Specifically, core SDG areas such as health service delivery, information systems, and health technologies are all likely to benefit from innovation around the adaptation of existing or design of new mHealth tools.

Leadership in the context of mHealth requires a willingness to take on new challenges. In this context, this means the goal of promoting equitable access to health service. This requires being prepared to adapt existing generic programs for repurposing and reflective practice and a willingness to reflect on what worked and how to improve. Finally, a clear, transparent communication across stakeholders is essential to ensuring sustainable, implementable mHealth programs.

This chapter describes three case studies where mHealth has been adapted for three distinct populations and purposes: (1) a healthy diet program for Hispanic populations in California, United States; (2) a smoking cessation program for Samoa, in the Pacific Islands region; and (3) a maternal health information program for multiple minority population families in New Zealand. These cases demonstrate the critical roles of innovation, flexibility in planning and goal setting, and transparent communications in leading these projects to successful outcomes.

Description of the Programs

The following section describes the mHealth initiatives in the Pacific Rim: United States (HealthyYouTXT), Samoa (TXTaofiTapaa), and New Zealand (TextMATCH). All three initiatives were designed to support behavior change by providing information and/or support, and all use text messages as the mode of delivery. Table 13.1 presents an overview of the three initiatives.

Table 13.1 Overview of the text-based initiatives

Intervention	Country	Population	Health target	Adaptation
HealthyYouTXT en Español	United States	Hispanic residents in the United States	Healthy dietary habits	Adapted from a general US population program
TXTTaofiTapaa	Samoa	Samoans and others living in Samoa	Smoking cessation	Adapted from a proven effective New Zealand program
TextMATCH	New Zealand	Māori, Pacific, South Asian, and Asian pregnant women, new mothers, and their families living in New Zealand	Maternal and child health, particularly healthy eating and physical activity	New program developed

Source: (Cameron et al., 2017; McCool, Umali, Tanielu, & Whittaker, 2017; Dobson, et al. 2017)

HealthyYouTXT en Español

HealthyYouTXT en Español is a culturally adapted Spanish version of HealthyYouTXT, a mHealth text messaging program developed by the US National Cancer Institute to promote healthy dietary practices. Guided by theory on motivation and behavior change, the program was designed to promote motivations to eat healthy foods while providing support, information and advice, reminders, and assistance in setting goals for healthy eating (Williams, Ryan, & Deci, 2015). HealthyYouTXT en Español was developed through transforming the English version of the program into a linguistically and culturally appropriate version for Spanish speakers living in the United States (Cameron et al., 2017). This process of adapting a generic or mainstream tool is key to improving equitable access to the benefits of mHealth, particularly to reach those who may benefit most.

The cultural adaptation process involved a three-stage, iterative process for translating and adapting the mHealth program. First, the messages went through multiple iterations of collaborative translations, independent back translations, and team discussions to enhance linguistic quality and adherence to thematic principles. Examples of thematic principles include infusion of familism (a value of prioritizing family over individual interests, which is widely held in Hispanic cultures) into messages, focus on culturally relevant foods (e.g., avocados, jicama, and salsas), and celebration. The next stage involved a sample of 109 Hispanic, Spanish-speaking residents of rural and non-rural communities who participated in a series of focus groups and surveys to provide both qualitative and quantitative data regarding the acceptability and cultural appropriateness of the messages. The final phase of adaptation involved a revision process to optimize the linguistic quality and cultural appropriateness of messages for Spanish speakers in rural, suburban, and urban communities.

A flexible and innovative leadership style was critical to bringing the HealthyYouTXT en Español program from the initial stages of development to implementation as a national resource freely available to all residents in the mainland United States. The endeavor involved working closely with the developers of the broader HealthyYouTXT program at the National Cancer Institute (NCI) to ensure that the HealthyYouTXT en Español met the specific requirements and constraints of the program technology, content structure, and agency regulations. Training and managing a team of health communication researchers and translators to meet these constraints throughout the program development process also took place. It also required flexibility and innovative problem solving to resolve issues revealed through the focus groups and surveys that did not fit within the existing program technology and content parameters. For example, the use of Spanish symbols emerged as critical to the acceptability of the program by Spanish speakers. Yet, the NCI's policy was to avoid using symbols since some users would have mobile phones that did not have the capacity to show symbols. The development of message principles to use alternative words instead of words with symbols and explaining this in the initial program descriptions to users overcame this problem.

TXTTaofiTapaa

TXTTaofiTapaa (TXT Stop Smoke) is a mobile phone-based smoking cessation intervention for Samoa. It was adapted from a New Zealand designed, text-based smoking cessation support program called STOMP (Rodgers et al., 2005; Bramley et al., 2005). With limited smoking cessation support available in Samoa, TXTTaofiTapaa presented an opportunity to provide smoking cessation support that was relatively affordable and readily available for Samoans who want to quit smoking. Initial exploratory research included focus groups with potential users (smokers) and ex-smokers. This included identifying the drivers to smoking and quitting, translating the message into the Samoan language, and then adapting the revised messages to reflect the cultural context of smoking in Samoa. During this period, researchers worked alongside the national government, a local nongovernment organization (NGO), telecommunications providers, and local stakeholders, including the World Health Organization (Samoa office). Each agency provided input into the content of messages and contributed to decisions about how the program would be pilot tested. After initial exploratory research among potential users, 92 messages were selected for the TXTTaofiTapaa program from the original database text messages of the STOMP program. In essence, a three-step cultural adaptation process was conducted including preliminary language translation (from English to Samoan), linguistic changes and cultural adaptation (with the Ministry of Health), and refinement of message content and delivery. The process of implementation of the program was contingent upon cooperation with the government and the telecommunications company. User engagement was also critical to allow users to become actively engaged in the design process to reflect their needs (e.g., timing and content of text messages), barriers (e.g., their peers), motivations (e.g., their family), and knowledge.

TextMATCH

The TextMATCH (Text messages for MATernal and Child Health) program was designed specifically to address the needs of four ethnic minority groups in Auckland, New Zealand: Māori (the indigenous population of New Zealand), Pacific, Asian, and South Asian residents (Dobson et al., 2017). The program was developed in collaboration with academics, representatives from public health, midwifery, nutrition, physical activity, Māori health promotion, primary care, and postnatal providers, as well as community organizations (Dobson et al., 2017). The final program, currently available in 16 different versions, takes into consideration culture, language, and relationship to the child (mother or other family member).

Initial formative work involved focus groups with target audiences, literature review, and review of national guidelines and publicly available resources. This led to the development of key messages and the identification of essential principles for ensuring cultural appropriateness (e.g., common foods and maternal health practices within each cultural group). Once confirmed, the contents of the messages were cultural adapted. Firstly, findings from the formative work were used to adapt all of the messages into the four distinct cultural versions incorporating the specific cultural factors/variables of the target groups. Secondly, the culturally adapted messages were fully translated into Te Reo Māori, Chinese, Korean, and Japanese. As requested by the target audiences, other versions were in English but incorporated greetings and other keywords in the appropriate languages (e.g., Hindi, Samoan, Tongan, Cook Island Maori, Tuvaluan, Tokelean). The community organizations from each of the cultural groups were involved throughout the development process to ensure the program was relevant for, and met the needs of, the target population. These groups reviewed and approved the final message sets, and translated messages were back translated to ensure the key messages remained correct (Dobson et al., 2017).

Outcomes

Adapting mHealth programs from one setting to another requires careful consideration of a number of factors. Our analysis of the outcomes of the three programs indicates that adaptation of mHealth tools for new populations required, at the very least, linguistic translation. This may be all that is needed to ensure a program becomes available (time and resources dispersed to delivery rather than refining), is accessible (able to be comprehended in local language or language of preference), and is based on principles of behavior change theory. Programs for diverse populations or programs being led in part by external agencies (particularly in LMICs) benefit from a deeper investment from all stakeholders to ensure that the program is culturally embedded within the health systems, rather than just culturally adapted.

In each of the three programs described, the cultural adaptation was conducted in addition to embedding the programs within their respective health systems. One of the main criticisms of mHealth innovations is that they infrequently move beyond the pilot phase, even if found to be acceptable and cost-effective. To address this challenge, we propose the following leadership elements as essential in process of adaptation and implementing mHealth initiatives.

Key Components of Leadership

- Conceptualizing and acting at scale: to ensure equity of opportunity to participate in the mHealth program. Throughout the mHealth initiatives described above, careful consideration of requirements needed for scaling up the program to the broader population (beyond the pilot sample) was essential. Elements of demonstrable leadership are constant reflection on access and equity. Despite the ubiquitous nature of mobile phones, keeping pace with developments in mobile access and literacy is important to mHealth in LMICS and underserved populations. Leadership is essential to provide options to make services accessible to their population—particularly to those who are disadvantaged or are not accessing traditional services.

- Leadership is innovation: in trialing new ideas, new modes of communication, reflecting on what works and what did not work in order to fine tune mHealth (as part of a wider health system intervention). It requires strong leadership to accept that business as usual is not going to achieve the gains that have been projected in several country, regional and global action plans. It takes some acceptance of risk and investment in new ways of doing things before it becomes completely clear whether this will pay off.

- Adaptation to context: is central to reflect the needs of the end-users and making necessary adjustments, in close consultation with those with the knowledge and connections with the end-users and those who will ultimately implement the mHealth program. While user engagement can vary in process and degree of complexity, as demonstrated by the three programs above, soliciting primary user input helps ensure that program design is not based on assumptions.

- Leadership at all levels: adaptation for a particular context requires leadership and commitment at the service level to ensure the program is going to be right for the respective community. Furthermore, leadership from the Ministry of Health or equivalent can help to demonstrate ownership and secure financial investment of the adapted program. Without this kind of commitment upfront, it can be difficult to get all the necessary stakeholders on-board. It is also critical for stakeholders to recognize that mobile health interventions should be designed to complement existing health system infrastructure.

Adapting a text message program is challenging when working cross-culturally and internationally. The TXTTaofiTapaa project, for example, underwent multiple iterations of independent linguistic adaptation. Although this process was useful, as the local government were implementing the program, they were the ones who needed to have the authority on translation and provide the final approval (McCool et al., 2017). Involving end-users, importantly, local end-users who represent the demographic groups who will be receiving the final messages are critical throughout. However, involving the key stakeholder—often, individuals who will be approving the rollout of any program—is equally important. Presenting a bank of near-complete messages to receive final approval prior to program initiation precludes a prime opportunity for relationship building. In other words, a text message program may be fastidiously designed, but without investment from key people within the local community, the perceived relevance of the program will be devalued.

Conclusion

This chapter has described three mHealth case studies highlighting the vital role of leadership in successful outcomes. Adapting mHealth programs from one setting to another requires careful consideration of a number of factors. Leadership qualities demonstrated through these mHealth adaptations include the drive to innovate, early engagement across the key stakeholders groups, and a willingness to reflect and learn. Effective leadership helps ensure that mHealth programs are accessible and relevant to their target population and that the innovative approach is embraced and accepted within the healthcare system.

References

Bramley, D., Riddell, T., Whittaker, R., Corbett, T., Lin, R. B., Wills, M., et al. (2005). Smoking cessation using mobile phone text messaging is as effective in Maori as non-Maori. *The New Zealand Medical Journal, 118*(1216), U1494.

Cameron, L. D., Durazo, A., Ramirez, A. S., Corona, C., Ultreras, M., & Piva, S. (2017). Cultural and linguistic adaptation of a healthy diet message interventions for Hispanic adults living in the United States. *Journal of Health Communication, 22,* 262–273.

Central Intelligence Agency (CIA). (2016). *CIA World Factbook.* Retrieved April 16, 2018, from https://www.cia.gov/library/publications/the-world-factbook/

Dobson, R., Whittaker, R., Bartley, H., Connor, A., Chen, R., Ross, M., et al. Development of a culturally tailored text message maternal health program: TextMATCH. *JMIR Mhealth Uhealth, 5*(4), e49. https://doi.org/10.2196/mhealth.7205

International Telecommunications Union. (2017). *Harnessing mobile technology to improve access to health care.* Retrieved April 16, 2018, from http://www.itu.int/en/ITU-D/Pages/TouchingLives.aspx?ItemID=13

McCool, J., Tanielu, H, Umali, E., Whittaker. (2017). Cross cultural adapation and translation of a teextbased mCessation programme in Samoa. JMIR uHealth and mHealth. In press

Rodgers, A., Corbett, T., Bramley, D., Riddell, T., Wills, M., Lin, R.-B., et al. (2005). Do u smoke after txt? Results of a randomised trial of smoking cessation using mobile phone text messaging. *Tobacco Control, 14,* 255–261.

Umali, E., McCool, J., & Whittaker, R. (2016). Possibilities and expectations for mHealth in the Pacific Islands: Insights from key informants. *JMIR mHealth and uHealth, 4*(1).

United Nations Development Programme (UNDP). (2016). *Human development report 2016.* Retrieved April 16, 2018, from http://hdr.undp.org/sites/default/files/2016_human_development_report.pdf.

Williams, G. C., Ryan, R. M., & Deci, E. L. (2015). Health-Care, Self-Determination Theory Questionnaire Packet. Retrieved March 1, 2015, from: http://www.selfdeterminationtheory.org/health-care-self-determinationtheory/

World Bank, (2018). World Bank Country Ranking. Low and middle income. https://data.worldbank.org/income-level/low-and-middle-income?view=chart. Accessed 1 August 2018.

World Health Organization. (2011). *mHealth: New horizons for health through mobile technologies: Second global survey on eHealth.* Retrieved April 16, 2018, from http://whqlibdoc.who.int/publications/2011/9789241564250_eng.pdf.

World Health Organization (WHO). (2015). *WHO statistical profile.* Retrieved April 16, 2018, from http://www.who.int/countries/en/.

Discussion Questions

1. Describe how mHealth can add support to the achievement of the SDGs and Universal Health Coverage.
2. Explain why adapting generic mHealth tools to each context is important.
3. Describe the three mHealth initiatives in the chapter and their distinctive characteristics in terms of context, end-user, behavior change objectives, and success elements.
4. Examine the potential benefits and risks of using an mHealth tool to deliver health services in low-resourced settings.

Follow-Up Reading

Chib, Arul, Michelle Helena van Velthoven, & Josip Car (2014). mHealth adoption in low-resource environments: A review of the use of mobile healthcare in developing countries. *Journal of Health Communication, 20*:1, 4–34. Available from https://doi.org/10.1080/10810730.2013.86 4735

International Telecommunications Union. *Harnessing mobile technology to improve access to health care.* Available from http://www.itu.int/en/ITU-D/Pages/TouchingLives. aspx?ItemID=13

Whittaker, R., Merry, S., Dorey, E., & Maddison, R. (2012). A development and evaluation process for mHealth interventions: examples from New Zealand. *Journal of Health Communication, 17*(sup1), 11–21.

World Health Organization (2016). *Monitoring and evaluating digital health interventions: A practical guide conducting research and assessment.* Geneva. Available from file:///C:/Users/jmcc092/Desktop/WHOmHealth-eng.pdf.

Glossary

2H2 2 Hari sebelum dan 2 Hari Sesudah = 2 days before and 2 days after delivery.
3D Dirty, dangerous, and difficult
Apps Smart phone applications
APRU Association of Pacific Rim Universities
CFO Commission on Filipino Overseas
Clery Act Jeanne Clery Disclosure of Campus Security Policy and Campus Crime Statistics Act
CPS American Cancer Society's Cancer Prevention Study
DFA Department of Foreign Affairs
DFA-OUMWA Department of Foreign Affairs – Office of the Undersecretary for Migrant Workers Affairs
DOLE Department of Labor and Employment
EAN Elder Abuse and Neglect-a single or repeated act, or lack of appropriate action, occurring within any relationship where there is an expectation of trust which causes harm or distress to an older person.
EPA United States Environmental Protection Agency
Familism A value of prioritizing family over individual interests.
FDIs Foreign direct investments
FGD Focus group discussion
FIRE Foundation for Individual Rights in Education
GNI Gross National Index
IDHS Indonesian Demographic Health Survey
IDI In-depth interview
ILSI Japan CHP International Life Sciences Institute Japan Center for Health Promotion
IMR Infant mortality rate
INDCs Intended Nationally Determined Contributions
IPCC Intergovernmental Panel on Climate Change
JICA Japan International Cooperation Agency
KCRR Korea Central Cancer Registry

© Springer Nature Switzerland AG 2019
M. Withers, J. McCool (eds.), *Global Health Leadership*,
https://doi.org/10.1007/978-3-319-95633-6

KIA Kesehatan Ibu dan Anak = Maternal and Child Health
Low- and Middle-income Countries (LMICs) LMIC is an economic or income grouping of countries by the World Bank and as of 2017, refers to countries with a per capita Gross National Income (GNI) between $1026 and $4035 using the World Bank Atlas method.
MAP Medical Aid Program
mHealth Mobile health
MMR Maternal Mortality Rate
MOH Ministry of Health
MOHW Ministry of Health and Welfare
NAAQS National Ambient Air Quality Standards
NCC National Cancer Center
NCI National Cancer Institute
NCIC National Cancer Information Center
NCSP National Cancer Screening Program
NGOs Non-governmental Organizations
NHI National Health Insurance
NIN National Institute of Nutrition
Non-communicable Diseases (NCDs) Non-communicable diseases (NCDs), also known as chronic diseases, are diseases that are not passed from person to person. They are of long duration and generally slow progression.
NRCO National Reintegration Center for Overseas Filipino Workers
NTT Nusa Tenggara Timur = East Nusa Tenggara, Indonesia
OAVS Overseas Absentee Voting Secretariat
OCR Office for Civil Rights
ODA Overseas development assistance
OFWs Overseas Filipino workers
Older Adults Generally, those aged 60 or more. In high income nations, the cut off is 65.
OWWA Overseas Workers Welfare Administration
PHN Primary Health Networks
Plain Packaging Tobacco packages that requires the removal of all company branding, including colors, imagery, corporate logos, and trademarks, only permitting the brand name in a standard font. The pack is then dominated by a large graphic health warning and quit smoking information.
PM Airborne particulate matter
POEA Philippine Overseas Employment Administration
POLOs Philippine Overseas Labor Offices
Puskesmas Pusat Kesehatan Masyarakat = Community Health Center
RCC Regional Cancer Center
Return on Investment (ROI) The economic benefit yielded from an initial financial investment.
RTD Round table discussion
SaVE Campus Sexual Violence Elimination Act
SCAR Student Coalition Against Rape

SDGs Sustainable Development Goals
SMS Short Message Service (text message)
SWAN Safe Water and Nutrition
TBA Traditional birth attendance
TextMATCH Text messages for MATernal and Child Health
TXTTaofiTapaa Text Stop Smoke
UNFCCC United Nations Framework Convention on Climate Change
UHC Universal Health Coverage
UN HDI United Nations Human Development Index
VAWA Violence Against Women Act
WASH Water, sanitation, and hygiene
WHO World Health Organization

Index

© Springer Nature Switzerland AG 2019
M. Withers, J. McCool (eds.), *Global Health Leadership*,
https://doi.org/10.1007/978-3-319-95633-6

Printed in the United States
By Bookmasters